The Consulting Therapist

A Guide for OTs and PTs in Schools

Barbara E. Hanft, M.A., OTR/L, FAOTA

Patricia A. Place, Ph.D.

Foreword by Susan K. Effgen, Ph.D., PT

Cover photography completed under contract by Thomas Veneklasen

Therapy Skill Builders®
a division of
The Psychological Corporation
555 Academic Court
San Antonio, Texas 78204-2498
1-800-228-0752

Reproducing Pages from This Book

As described below, some of the pages in this book may be reproduced for instructional or administrative use (not for resale). To protect your book, make a photocopy of each reproducible page. Then use that copy as a master for photocopying.

Special thanks to cover models Justen Fastje, Ben Huntington, Danielle Lee, Jesse Niwa, and Stephanie Schultz.

Therapy Skill Builders®
a division of
The Psychological Corporation
555 Academic Court
San Antonio, Texas 78204-2498
1-800-228-0752

ISBN 0761643656

10 9 8 7 6

Printed in the United States of America

Dedication

To Karen and Ryan, who teach us all about living and learning.

About the Authors

Barbara E. Hanft, M.A., OTR/L, FAOTA is a Faculty Emeritus of Sensory Integration International and has more than 20 years of experience providing pediatric occupational therapy and family counseling services in special education, mental health, and early intervention settings. She received the M.A. degree in counseling psychology from the University of California at Santa Barbara. Recognized as a Fellow of the American Occupational Therapy Association (AOTA) for her leadership and advocacy in pediatrics, Ms. Hanft has worked in the national offices of AOTA and lobbied Congress and the U.S. Department of Education to amend special education laws and create early intervention services. She has developed a broad range of continuing education programs for AOTA, including a nationally recognized program taught by parent/professional teams to promote family-centered care. At present, Ms. Hanft is a developmental consultant and a respected author and trainer on topics related to early intervention and school-based therapy.

Patricia A. Place, Ph.D., is a developmental psychologist. She received the M.Ed. degree in early childhood special education from the University of North Carolina at Chapel Hill and the Ph.D. degree in child study from Tufts University, Medford, Massachusetts. A recognized expert in special and preschool education, Dr. Place has provided training and consultation to educators and administrators across the country in the areas of policy development and research, interdisciplinary collaboration, and family and child advocacy. Her own classroom experience includes teaching in public school and hospital settings and working closely with therapists and other related service providers. Dr. Place has directed the National Forum on Children and Families at the National Academy of Sciences in Washington, DC, and currently is the principal investigator of Project Begin, an early intervention initiative conducted by the Developmental Disabilities Prevention Unit of the U.S. Centers for Disease Control.

Contents

Acknowledgments

We are indebted to Susan Effgen, Ph.D., PT; Jean Linder, M.A., OTR/L; and Kathy Sack, RPT, for their thoughtful review and insightful comments during the preparation of this text.

Foreword

The progression from direct service provider to consultant requires more than expertise in developmental assessment and treatment. Therapists must also understand the roles and responsibilities of the consultant, be able to work successfully with teams of families and professionals from many disciplines, understand the milieu and classroom etiquette, and be especially comfortable with their own knowledge and skills to be able to share them easily without being threatening. Entry-level therapy programs prepare graduates to practice, but experience is required before the therapist is ready to provide effective consultation. Therefore, therapists usually rely on their day-to-day experiences and perhaps continuing education to learn the skills necessary to become a successful consultant.

Barbara Hanft and Patricia Place have made it easy to learn about consultation specific to occupational and physical therapists in education settings, filling a major void in the literature. The authors' years of experience are evidenced by their insight as to what is necessary to become a successful and welcome member of an educational team. They understand that a therapist must appreciate the philosophy, roles, and responsibilities of the classroom teacher and the unique needs of the child with a disability in the school setting. They carefully guide the reader through the requirements necessary to provide educationally relevant consultative services.

The Consulting Therapist will be a valuable reference to all therapists working in education settings. The authors should be commended for undertaking such an important task. Occupational and physical therapists will appreciate the authors' comprehensive review of the literature on school-based therapy. Current best practice in pediatric therapy in any setting requires that we consider how to work collaboratively with professional colleagues and family members to expand the impact of our direct therapeutic intervention.

The ultimate beneficiaries of this work will be the children with disabilities and their families, whose lives are enriched and made easier by appropriate and coordinated educational services.

Susan K. Effgen, Ph.D., PT
Director, Pediatric Physical Therapy
Medical College of Pennsylvania and Hahnemann University
Philadelphia, Pennsylvania

Preface

We believe that occupational and physical therapists should include collaborative consultation in every intervention plan developed for children with special needs, whether the setting is a school, home, hospital, or clinic. Through collaborative consultation, therapists assist other people—family members, educators, classroom aides, child-care providers, even other therapists—to help children achieve desired outcomes. Consultation and direct service models provide distinctly different, but equally important, ways for therapists to contribute their expertise to enhance children's performance. In their professional preparation and continuing education programs, therapists learn how to provide direct intervention, but very little formal instruction is offered regarding how to become an effective consulting therapist.

The primary reason for writing this book is to focus on the art and science of using collaborative consultation effectively to benefit children and families in school settings. Providing effective consultation requires unique skills that most therapists do not learn during the course of their professional education but find they need once they begin working. Our goals are to explain the process of collaborative consultation and show through stories and vignettes how it can be used effectively in school settings.

The Consulting Therapist is based on the extensive school experiences we each have had in our respective roles as therapist and educator working with students who have special needs. In addition, we have benefitted enormously from our participation in various consulting relationships as both the consultant and consultee. We have organized this material to reflect our view that therapists must provide intervention within a specific context; in this case, collaborative consultation within an education setting.

While reading *The Consulting Therapist,* several points are important to keep in mind. First, family members are an essential part of the school team, not just the signers of their child's IEP; therefore, the word *team* always includes both professionals and families. Second, the vignettes focus on preschool and elementary students since this is the age group that the majority of school-based therapists serve. However, our points about collaborative consultation can be applied to any age group of students. Third, our material applies to all therapists working in the schools, whether they call themselves consultants and provide contract services or are employed by the schools as staff therapists, since all therapists should include collaborative consultation as an integral component of their intervention. Finally, we use the term *consulting therapist* throughout the book to include both occupational and physical therapists and do not distinguish between the professions since we believe the process of collaborative consultation is the same for each.

We hope to convince you that effective school-based therapy always includes consultation and to inspire you to develop your collaborative skills to help students with special needs fit in and learn at school.

Barbara E. Hanft, M.A., OTR/L, FAOTA
Patricia A. Place, Ph.D.

Chapter 1 lays the foundation for understanding consultation as an essential service model in the school system by highlighting:

- the role of occupational and physical therapists in the schools, as mandated by federal legislation and regulations, court cases, and due process hearings
- differences between the traditional medical and education intervention models
- myths about consultation
- characteristics and benefits of effective collaborative consultation

Chapter 1

Working and Consulting in the School System

Collaborative consultation is becoming increasingly important as professionals in all walks of life attempt to cope effectively in a rapidly changing, increasingly complex society.

Phillips and McCullough 1990

School reform has many advocates from diverse sectors of society, including education, government, business, and rehabilitation. One critical reform focuses on providing consultation for students whose needs are not met by existing regular or special education programs (Phillips and McCullough 1990; Peck, Killen, and Baumgart 1989). Occupational and physical therapists have also called for expanding direct service to include consultation with families and educators to serve students with special needs in self-contained and general education classrooms (Fisher 1994; Rainforth, York, and MacDonald 1992; Dunn and Campbell 1991; Effgen 1994; Hanft 1989). Some studies have found consultation to be as beneficial as direct service in promoting student outcomes (Dunn 1990; Giangreco 1986; Schulte, Osborne, and McKinney 1990; Miller and Sabatino 1978). In addition, educators have indicated their preference in many situations for in-class, rather than "pull-out," assistance from therapists and other specialists (Meyers, Gelzheiser, and Yelich 1991; Cole et al. 1989). Finally, the inclusion of children with disabilities in regular classrooms has highlighted the need for collaborative consultation among special educators, regular educators, and therapists (Idol, Nevin, and Paolucci-Whitcomb 1994; Dunn 1991).

Despite the recognized benefits of collaborating with educational staff, the art of consultation in schools remains a challenge for most therapists. Basic professional education prepares occupational and physical therapists to work with individuals across the life cycle and does not universally emphasize pediatric assessment and intervention (Spake 1994; AOTA Pediatric Task Force 1989). Even within pediatric courses and fieldwork, there is a limited focus on school system practice (Effgen 1988). In addition, very few university students or practicing clinicians receive formal training in the art of consultation; direct, "hands-on" service is still the primary model taught in basic professional training as well as continuing education for therapists in practice.

As a result, therapists as well as teachers are generally taught to work in clinics or their own classrooms with children, rather than consulting with one another. They often learn to consult "on the fly" during periodic interactions with one another throughout the school day. *The Consulting Therapist* focuses on how to provide occupational and physical therapy services in an education setting using a collaborative consultation model. As every school-based therapist knows, working in an educational setting is a very different experience from working in a medical setting. Likewise, consulting with a teacher or family member is not the same as providing hands-on intervention to a student.

Therapists' Involvement in the Educational System

A review of how therapists became involved in the educational system provides a basis for understanding their role as consulting therapists. Occupational and physical therapists began working in the school system in significant numbers after 1935, when federal grants to the states created Crippled Children's Services (CCS) under the Maternal and Child Health Program of the Social Security Act. Initially, services were provided to children with orthopedic and neurological problems, particularly due to polio. During the 1940s and 1950s, occupational and physical therapists were hired by county CCS clinics to work in public schools to provide direct service to children with cerebral palsy, polio, muscular dystrophy, and other orthopedic problems. Therapists often worked in separate schools just for children with physical or mental disabilities (Fisher 1994; Komich 1991).

According to the U.S. Congress, during the 1960s and early 1970s, one million children were denied the opportunity to attend public school because they were considered uneducable (Individuals with Disabilities Education Act, 20 U.S.C. 33, Sec. 1400). The majority of these children had severe and profound disabilities in several developmental domains. Many were not able to talk, walk, or learn through standard educational practices of the day. Therapists served students with significant motor and self-help delays who were able, or allowed, to attend school. During this time, therapists saw their primary duty as providing direct service to students in the school environment, replicating the clinic and hospital practice they were trained to provide. Establishing a referral system, buying or making equipment, evaluating and treating students, and orienting education personnel to therapy services was a full-time job. Little time was left to ponder how to provide educationally relevant therapy, either through direct service or consultation.

During the early 1970s, two major judicial decisions (Pennsylvania Association for Retarded Children v. Commonwealth of Pennsylvania; Mills v. DC Board of Education), affirmed that all children had a right to a public education. At the same time, Congress passed the Education for the Handicapped Act (EHA) and added significant amendments in 1975 with the Education for All Handicapped Children Act (P.L. 94-142) requiring states to provide special education and related services, including occupational and physical therapy, to all eligible children between the ages of 6 and 18 to 21 years. Subsequent amendments to the EHA in 1986 offered states the incentives to lower the eligibility age for special education and related services to three years and created a discretionary grant program for statewide, interagency early intervention services for infants and toddlers with special needs. In 1991, the EHA's title was changed to the Individuals with Disabilities Education Act (IDEA), recognizing the importance of identifying children as individuals before identifying their disability.

The number of children with disabilities served by therapists in school settings increased dramatically as states began implementing these laws. When P.L. 94-142 was first passed in 1975, approximately 5% of occupational therapists worked in the school system; in 1991 that figure increased to 18% and the school system became the single largest employer of occupational therapy personnel, nudging out hospitals by only a fraction of a percent. By 1993, approximately 15,000 (33%) members of the American Occupational Therapy Association (AOTA) worked primarily with children and adolescents (AOTA 1993). Approximately 10% of the members of the American Physical Therapy Association (APTA) surveyed in 1993 specialized in pediatrics and almost half of those practitioners reported the schools as their primary work setting (APTA 1994; Sweeney, Heriza, and Markowitz 1994).

As P.L. 94-142 was implemented, therapists recognized the stark difference between their medical model training and practice in the educational system. The AOTA and APTA responded to therapists' needs for assistance in school-based practice. In 1974, a pediatric section was formally recognized by the APTA and the school system became the prominent employment setting for pediatric section members (Sweeney, Heriza, and Markowitz 1994). In 1980, the AOTA disseminated a federally supported inservice program for school-based therapists, entitled *TOTEMS: Training Occupational Therapy Educational Management in the Schools* (Gilfoyle and Hays 1980). In addition, both AOTA and APTA have published school guidelines, which are currently undergoing revision (Martin 1990; Chandler, Dunn, and Rourk 1989). Two other resources highlighting school system practice and consultation in the classroom were published by AOTA as self-study courses for occupational and physical therapists (Royeen 1991, 1992). In addition, the AOTA established a special interest section for school-based therapists in 1993.

The Role of Therapists in the Schools

There are many points of contrast between practice in education and traditional medical settings (see table 1.1, page 4). In the traditional medical model, which has undergone extensive restructuring over the past 10 years with health-care reform, pediatric therapists are taught to help children improve their skills and achieve maximum function in sensory, motor, self-help, perceptual, and adaptive behavior domains through their respective disciplinary modalities and activities. The consumer of services is a "patient" who is sick, injured, or was born with a disability. Therapy is provided to minimize the impact of this injury or disability and to maximize skill and independence in whatever environment and role the "patient" encounters in daily life activities in home, school, and other community environments. The majority of the cost of therapy services for children is covered by Medicaid, private health insurance, and out-of-pocket payments by parents.

Table 1.1
A Comparison of Medical and Educational Models

Component	Traditional Medical Model	Regular/Special Education Model
View of consumer	patient who is ill from disease, injury, or congenital anomaly	student who can learn curriculum
View of disability	physical/mental condition from disease or injury	1 of 13 impairments affecting learning (as defined in IDEA)
Goal of intervention	heal/cure	impart knowledge, enhance learning and development
Primary services	diagnosis, drugs, surgery	classroom instruction, special education, and related services
Primary providers	physicians and nurses	educators, special educators, and related service providers in special education
Responsibility for decisions	physician	educators, family, and related service providers
Focus of assessment	patient health status and symptoms	student readiness and academic achievement, learning impairments
Intervention plan	treatment plan to cure illness or heal injury	curriculum to acquire skill by grade, IEP for special education
Access to services	varies by location and ability to pay	guaranteed by law, at age 3 for special education
Payment for services	insurance and out-of-pocket	local property taxes, state and federal taxes
Service site	physician's office, hospital, clinic	public and private schools
Frequency of contact	episodic, initiated when ill or injured	daily
Benefit from therapy	rehabilitation: maximum skills and independence	assist student to benefit from special education

Therapists who attempt to implement their traditional medical model training are frequently challenged when they work in the public schools, whose mission is to teach students a specified curriculum, usually defined by grade and geographic location. Public schools are mandated to provide free, appropriate education to all children with disabilities who need special education and related services. Under IDEA provisions, students with disabilities who receive special education are entitled to occupational or physical therapy only if it will help them benefit from their special education program. Therapy is tied to special education, so it is defined as a *related* service. The education team, including parents and caregivers, can include necessary physical or occupational therapy services on the student's Individualized

Education Program (IEP), the legal document describing a student's special education placement and related services. While these services must be provided at no charge to families, with their permission private insurance and Medicaid can be billed to cover physical or occupational therapy.

The role of occupational and physical therapists in the schools is further defined by specific provisions under IDEA that address eligibility for special education and related services, scope of practice, IEP components, and provisions for educating students in the least restrictive environment (see table 1.2). The pivotal term for understanding medically based versus school-based therapy is *appropriate*. Therapists using a medical model may mistakenly assume that appropriate physical or occupational therapy intervention is equivalent to helping students achieve their maximum level of independence in the school environment. In a landmark decision handed down in 1982 (Board of Education v. Rowley), the Supreme Court concluded that Congress intended to grant students with disabilities access to educational opportunities by ensuring that they could go to public school, not that they receive the best education or one designed to help them reach maximum potential (Turnbull 1986). The Supreme Court also affirmed that children with disabilities were entitled to personalized instruction with sufficient support services, such as physical or occupational therapy, to permit them to benefit educationally from that instruction.

Table 1.2
Legal Mandates for Related Services under IDEA

Provision in Part B Regulations (34 C.F.R. Parts 300 and 301)	Implication for Practice
Children with disabilities	
Sec. 300.7(a)(1) . . . children evaluated . . . as having the following impairments: mental retardation, hearing including deafness, speech or language, visual including blindness, serious emotional disturbance, orthopedic, autism, traumatic brain injury, other health impairments, specific learning disabilities, deaf-blindness, or multiple disabilities, and who because of those impairments need special education and related services	According to IDEA, a child does not have a disability unless he or she needs special education.
Sec. 300.7 (a)(2)(I) children aged 3-5 years may . . . include children who are experiencing developmental delays, as defined by the State and measured by appropriate diagnostic instruments and procedures, in one or more of the following areas: physical, cognitive, communication, social or emotional or adaptive development	Preschool children may not have to receive a diagnostic label other than "developmental delay."
Related Services Sec. 300.16(a) . . . means transportation and other supportive services required to assist a child with a disability to benefit from special education, and includes . . . physical and occupational therapy . . .	Since occupational and physical therapy are mandated under IDEA, school districts must provide therapy, but only for children with disabilities who need therapy to benefit from special education.

Table 1.2 (continued)

Provision in Part B Regulations (34 C.F.R. Parts 300 and 301)	Implication for Practice
Definitions of Service Physical therapy Sec. 330.16(b)(7) . . . means services provided by a qualified physical therapist Occupational therapy Sec. 330.16(b)(5) includes: (i). improving, developing or restoring functions impaired or lost through illness, injury or deprivation (ii). improving ability to perform tasks for independent functioning when functions are impaired or lost (iii). preventing, through early intervention, initial or further impairment or loss of function	Definitions of practice do not address how services are provided, thus they neither recommend nor disallow consultation over direct service.
Content of IEP Sec. 300.346(a) 1. child's present level of educational performance 2. annual goals and short-term objectives 3. specific special education and related services to be provided and the extent child will participate in regular education programs 4. projected dates for initiation of services and anticipated duration of services 5. appropriate objective criteria and evaluation procedures and schedules for determining, on at least an annual basis, whether the short-term instructional objectives are being achieved	Physical and/or occupational therapy must be included on a student's IEP in order to receive therapy services. The IEP is the official document for deciding whether an education plan is appropriate for a specific student.
Least restrictive environment Sec. 300.550 (b) Each public agency shall ensure: (1) that to the extent appropriate, children with disabilities, including children in public or private institutions or other care facilities, are educated with children who are nondisabled; and (2) that special classes, separate schooling or the removal of children with disabilities from the regular educational environment, occurs only when the nature or severity of the disability is such that education in regular classes with the use of supplementary aids and services cannot be achieved satisfactorily	Therapy should be provided in a manner that facilitates the integration of students with disabilities with their peers.

While the IDEA established that occupational and physical therapy are related services that should be provided to eligible students in special education, nothing is said in the law or regulations about *how* these services are to be provided. However, program requirements and student rights have been clarified by administrative decisions in due process hearings at the state and local education levels. Some of these decisions describe when physical or occupational therapy consultation is appropriate for an individual student (see table 1.3). Our review of due process decisions indicates that consultation is an appropriate service model for an individual student when:

- school personnel are qualified to implement the therapists' suggestions
- the student's educational needs (benefit from special education) would be met as well or better than through direct service
- therapy can be provided in the least restrictive manner in classrooms and regular school activities

Table 1.3
Examples of Due Process Decisions Affecting Occupational and Physical Therapy Consultation in the Classroom

Issue	Decision	Analysis	Reference
School proposes consultative physical and occupational therapy for 3½-year-old boy with Down syndrome who has fine and gross motor delays; parents request direct service.	Direct service denied and consultation one hour per week by PT and OT recommended.	Direct service to maximize student's potential is not required; direct services are more restrictive than consultative; teachers do not have the expertise to meet student's motor needs; they can be met through consultation.	1986-87 *Education for the Handicapped Law Review,* 508:255-259
After one year of direct service, school proposes that consultation by OT to classroom teacher be provided to student in class for mild mental handicaps; parents request direct service to continue.	Direct service two times per week awarded.	While therapy provided by a teacher under supervision of a licensed therapist meets state requirements in Indiana, the school failed to show that the necessary therapy identified on the IEP could be appropriately delivered for this student via consultation.	1982 *Education for the Handicapped Law Review,* 504:222-224
School proposes OT consultation one time per month with adaptive physical education teacher for 6-year-old boy with fine and gross motor delays and visual-motor deficits; parents request direct service.	Consultation one time per month with adaptive PE teacher awarded.	Given the progress made in achieving IEP objectives through activities provided by the regular and resource teachers, the student does not require direct service.	1982 *Education for the Handicapped Law Review,* 504:349-351

It is important to understand that due process hearings at the state and local education agencies affect an individual child and are not automatically applicable to all students unless included in law or regulations, incorporated in court decisions, or written into formal federal and state policies. Just because occupational or physical therapy consultation is found to be an appropriate service model to meet the education needs of one student in a due process hearing does not mean all other students should receive therapy via a consultative model. Moreover, while due process decisions have supported the provision of consultative services, in some cases decisions have been rendered favoring direct service over consultation. This happens when educational staff cannot meet the student's IEP objectives through consultation from therapists (1984-85, *Education for the Handicapped Law Report,* DEC. 504:222-224) or when direct service had already resulted in substantially documented progress (1985-86, Education for the Handicapped Law Report, DEC. 507:197-199). The bottom line is that consultation is a viable service option when chosen to meet the educational needs of a specific student.

Myths about Consultation in the School System

Three prevalent myths concerning consultation in the schools, reflect administrators' and therapists' misconceptions about school-based practice:

- Therapists can dramatically increase their case loads through consultation.
- When consulting in the classroom, therapists train teachers to do physical and occupational therapy.
- Consultation can always substitute for direct service.

The first myth, that therapists can greatly increase their case loads, is often the administrative answer to the shortage of therapists in the school. Many administrators seize upon consultation as a service model, hoping to significantly increase educators' and therapists' case loads. Effective consultation takes as much time as direct service (Dunn 1991; Idol-Maestas and Ritter 1985). Therapists must analyze the student's performance in the educational context, clarify roles and expectations of educational team members, and assist with developing and evaluating desired outcomes and interventions for students with disabilities.

The second myth, that consultation results in the teacher doing therapy, comes from therapists' basic misunderstanding about when and why to use consultation. Too often consultation is chosen by therapists or dictated by administrators *before* a student's educational needs are determined. When this occurs, therapists may ask teachers to carry out what they would have done had they provided direct service. In essence, the therapist is asking the teacher to be the therapist, instead of making recommendations that fit the teacher's role and function. Educators have their own responsibilities (teaching the curriculum) and are not trained as occupational and physical therapists. Therapists, however, can and should assist educators with modifying instruction and implementing appropriate activities so that students acquire the necessary skills and behaviors to learn and behave at school.

The third myth is that consultation can always substitute for direct intervention, especially if the therapist recommends activities for the classroom. In our experience, consultation can be as, or more, effective than direct service when it is chosen specifically as the service model for helping a student reach a specific outcome. Frequently, a student can benefit from a combination of direct service and consultation; it is not always an either/or decision. While it is our belief that direct service in the schools should always be accompanied by consultation with educational staff and family members, the reverse is not always true. Not all students need direct service to enhance their performance in the school setting. At a due process hearing, an occupational therapist clarified the importance of consultation to adapt the class environment for a young child with hemiparesis placed in a regular preschool:

> . . . I would say providing therapy as an adjunct to a preschool program would be best for her and it is not just the laying on of hands for one hour a week that is going to give [her] the best. It is putting her in an environment with other children and looking at the deficits, trying to minimize the deficit by adapting the environment around her so that she can keep up with other children.
>
> 1984-85 *Education for the Handicapped Law Report,* DEC. 506:101, p. 102

It is critical that the desired outcomes for the student be identified *before* deciding that occupational or physical therapy is needed or *before* choosing a service model for providing therapy. Consultation can be effective whenever the therapist and team decide it is the best method to improve a student's performance by adapting the school environment and materials or setting up classroom programs for other team members to implement. Consultation will not be effective when provided to compensate for personnel shortages. When chosen inappropriately, families and educators view consultation as a second-rate substitute for direct service. The following scenario illustrates how these three myths about consultation affect one therapist's attempts to serve the children on her case load by working with the teacher in the classroom.

Ravi, a third-grader with mild cerebral palsy, tires easily during paper-and-pencil tasks. After writing only three sentences, he slumps in his seat, rests his head on his desk, and looks out the window. Meagan is an itinerant therapist who was asked to consult with Ravi's teacher, Mr. Darvone. Meagan recognized the effect of poor fine motor skills, low muscle tone, and wrist instability on Ravi's posture and pencil grip as contributing factors in his dislike for any task involving handwriting.

Meagan feels Ravi would benefit from direct intervention but has been told by her supervisor to add 15 students to her case load by consulting just once per month (myth 1). So she recommends to Mr. Darvone, the classroom teacher, that Ravi do some of the exercises she would have done in direct service, including pulling and pushing activities using elastic therapy bands and putty to improve forearm and wrist stability (myth 2).

She asks Mr. Darvone to do these exercises twice per day, once before language arts in the morning and once in the afternoon before science when Ravi records the results of his nature observations. Meagan explains in simple language how the exercises will improve Ravi's posture and grip and make handwriting less tiring. She even goes one step further and makes up a chart for Mr. Darvone to check off with Ravi when he completes his exercises (myth 3).

Why is Meagan surprised when Mr. Darvone fails to implement her recommendations? Several problems are evident. First, Meagan never discussed her observations and conclusions with Mr. Darvone, nor did she ask for his ideas as to why Ravi disliked handwriting tasks. Meagan also needed to address Mr. Darvone's educational outcomes for Ravi: that he complete his written assignments within a specified time period. Meagan wanted to see Ravi in individual therapy to improve his muscle tone and joint stability. Since she did not have room on her case load to treat Ravi herself, she recommended some of her therapy exercises for Mr. Darvone to carry out in the classroom. Meagan needed to explain the relationship of Ravi's immature grasp of the pencil on his writing speed and recommend adaptations, such as using a slantboard and special pencil grip that would help Ravi compensate for poor wrist stability and an inefficient grasp. By increasing Ravi's skill in handling his pencil, Meagan could address the educational goal of completing class assignments within a specified length of time. During her discussions with Mr. Darvone, Meagan could also suggest appropriate targets for how long Ravi can reasonably be expected to write before fatiguing.

Finally, Meagan presented her recommendations to Mr. Darvone as a *fait accompli,* without asking if it was possible for him to carry them out. Although she tried to gear her recommendations for a small space in the classroom, Meagan assumed that because she could carry them out, so could Mr. Darvone. Meagan never looked at Ravi's daily schedule to find naturally occurring times to provide the kind of intervention she felt would be beneficial.

Let us suppose that Meagan realizes that she can help Ravi achieve the stated educational outcomes and improve his wrist stability through classroom consultation alone or by using a combination of both direct service and consultation. She begins to wonder about using consultation for other students and is intrigued by a colleague's comment that he provides integrated therapy right in the classroom and never sees students in "pull-out" (a separate therapy space). Like most school-based therapists, Meagan begins thinking about all the different terms she has heard recently to describe school-based therapy services and wonders just where consultation fits in.

Collaborative Consultation in Schools

Consultation is a process of providing therapy services to enhance student performance primarily by working with classroom teachers, families, and other team members. This process is an important component of the following models identified in the literature:

Integrated programming or therapy. Working with team members to provide occupational and physical therapy within naturally occurring contexts throughout the school day (York, Rainforth, and Giangreco 1990)

Monitoring or management. Developing a student program that is implemented by team members in the school environment with ongoing supervision from a therapist (Chandler, Dunn, and Rourk 1989; Effgen 1994)

Consultation to other team members. Recommending teaching strategies, equipment adaptation, or modifications of the classroom environment (Dunn 1991)

Obviously, these models cover overlapping roles and functions. Some of the therapy literature regarding school system practice refers to consultation as infrequent service of short duration to educators (Rainforth, York, and MacDonald 1992) or the service model of choice "when skills need to be generalized to natural environments, or when the environment can be adapted to support more functional behavior" (Dunn 1991).

Since our objective is to focus on how to work effectively with others to enhance student performance, we use the term *consultation* to refer to the collaborative process that occurs in integrated therapy, monitoring, or brief and ongoing interaction with teachers. Even when a therapist provides direct service in a "pull-out" model, we believe that ongoing consultation with teachers and other team members should be provided to ensure that therapy recommendations are incorporated in meaningful ways in a student's daily school activities.

Three critical elements support effective consultation: dynamic interaction over time, respectful relationships, and collaborative efforts to reach common ground. The first element, interaction over time, highlights that consultation is a voluntary, dynamic process between therapists and other team members. Effective consultation takes time; rarely is it effectively provided in only one short meeting among therapists and parents or educators. It also must be voluntary. It is very difficult to elicit cooperation from educators or parents when their participation or support for consultation is involuntary or undesired. Likewise, therapists who prefer working with students themselves are not likely to pay enough attention to the interaction among the adult team members that is so crucial to effective consultation.

The second element, respectful relationships, recognizes the special knowledge and experience of all participants in the consultation process. Educators have indicated their preference for a collaborative model of consultation, expressed in terms of, "Let's meet as equals on this," rather than, "You tell me what to do" (Babcock and Pryzwansky 1983; Pryzwansky and White 1983). When the consultant elicits rather than presents information, team members are less likely to resist recommendations and more likely to suggest other ideas to try (Bergan and Neumann 1980).

Collaborative efforts among therapists, educators, other specialists, and family members who agree to work together toward a common goal is the final element. Joint identification of the student's abilities and educational needs leads to the establishment of a common ground upon which to base goals and recommendations. One of the primary mistakes therapists make when they begin consulting is to assume that their views and goals are shared by teachers or parents. Consultation is an indirect model of working through another person to help the student function in the school environment. It is not a method to persuade others to implement your goals. As you will read in the next chapters, consulting therapists must understand what other team members want the student to learn or achieve. Naturally, as part of the consultation process, therapists' views and suggestions for outcomes and goals must also be expressed and discussed. All parties involved in the process have an equally important, yet different, knowledge and experience base.

A classic definition of collaborative consultation developed by educators is equally useful for therapists:

> . . . collaborative consultation is an interactive process that enables teams of people with diverse expertise to generate creative solutions to mutually defined problems. The outcome is enhanced, altered and produces solutions that are different from those that the individual team member would produce independently. The major outcome of collaborative consultation is to provide

comprehensive and effective programs for students with special needs within the most appropriate context, thereby enabling them to achieve maximum constructive interaction with their nonhandicapped peers.

Idol, Paolucci-Whitcomb, and Nevin 1987

Benefits of Consultation

Four major benefits arise from using consultation to provide school-based occupational and physical therapy:

Makes effective use of available personnel. Consultation expands the impact of direct service so that students receive the added benefits of the physical and occupational therapists' recommendations throughout the school day. By understanding teachers' responsibilities, the consulting therapist can plan interventions to help them enhance student skills and behavior.

Supports inclusion and the IDEA mandate for providing services in the least restrictive environment. Consulting therapists can integrate their specialized approaches and knowledge by providing intervention during regular school activities and in spaces such as the classroom, lunchroom, or gym rather than separate therapy areas isolated from the flow of the daily school routine.

Builds skills of other professionals. Consulting therapists can enhance the knowledge and skills of other team members and model desired intervention so that others learn different ways to interact with and teach children.

Enhances resources for problem solving. Collaborative consultation is based on an exchange of information between partners who have different, but equally important, experiences and knowledge. By facilitating the pooling of this talent, consulting therapists can promote the development of creative programs to identify and achieve appropriate educational outcomes for each student.

Conclusion

We have highlighted how therapists became involved as essential providers in the school system and have discussed the differences in practice between the education and traditional medical models. In describing the role of physical and occupational therapists in the schools, we emphasized the legal provisions in federal law and regulations that affect how therapists provide intervention in the schools. We have also provided some insight from due process hearings regarding how consultation can become a viable service model when students need occupational or physical therapy to benefit from special education. Finally, our description of collaborative consultation in the schools as an indirect process of working though educators and family members to enhance student performance is based on three critical factors:

- dynamic, voluntary interaction and relationships
- respect for the knowledge and experience of consultants and consultees
- collaborative effort to identify common ground, including perspectives, goals and objectives, and strategies for intervention

Selected Readings

Long, T., Ed. 1994. *Pediatric Physical Therapy* 6(3):105-178.

This issue of *Pediatric Physical Therapy* is devoted to celebrating the 20th anniversary of the establishment of the APTA Section on Pediatrics. Many of the articles discuss the role of the physical therapist in schools, the effect of special education legislation on practice, and changes in pediatric theory and practice.

Phillips, V., and L. McCullough. 1990. Consultation-based programming: Instituting the collaborative ethic in schools. *Exceptional Children* 56(4):291-304.

This article discusses the principles that support consultation in school settings and identifies factors that maximize its potential for success. Written for educators, the article provides an important look at the climate necessary for effective consultation by any professional working in an education setting.

Royeen, C., Ed. 1991. *School-based practice for related services.* Rockville, MD: American Occupational Therapy Association.

This excellent self-study course was designed for occupational and physical therapists and speech-language pathologists who work in schools. Nine lessons address topics including IDEA provisions, how to write functional goals, consulting as a process, working in the education system, and gaining control of documentation. Each lesson is accompanied by commentary from an expert OT, PT, or SLP who relates the topic specifically to that profession.

Turnbull, H. R. 1986. *Free appropriate public education: The law and children with disabilities.* Denver: Love.

This book provides an excellent discussion of the six major principles of the Individuals with Disabilities Education Act: right to education, testing and placement, individualized and appropriate education, least restrictive environment, procedural due process, and parent participation. Judicial decisions affecting special education and related services are also reviewed.

Chapter 2 discusses the relationship of educationally relevant services to the process of collaborative consultation by:

- describing educational relevance as it applies to physical and occupational therapy
- illustrating how therapy can enhance student performance in the school setting through the use of collaborative consultation
- identifying the educational outcomes and indicators of problems for typical therapy domains

Chapter 2

Educationally Relevant Consultation

A humorous example of how a therapist's clinical perspective can obscure meaning was reported by a program director who accompanied his staff occupational therapist to a parent conference. After a long explanation of why the child needed R-O-M for his R-U-E, the mother finally asked what an R-U-E was. When the therapist answered "right upper extremity," the mother replied that in her family it was called an "A-R-M."

Feinberg 1994

Simply stated, educational relevance refers to whether occupational and physical therapy services, whatever their form, help explain and enhance student performance in school. In order to provide educationally relevant services, therapists must have knowledge of the students' abilities and performance in the educational environment, whether in a preschool setting, resource room, or general education classroom. This does not mean that physical and occupational therapists should address only academic subjects; rather, they must look at how a student's basic sensory, motor, and perceptual skills and adaptive behavior provide a foundation for or impede learning. A clarification of IEP requirements from the U.S. Department of Education issued in 1981 describes the areas that are appropriate to include on a student's IEP:

> The statement of present levels of educational performance will be different for each child with a disability. Thus, determinations about the content of the statement for an individual child are matters that are left to the discretion of participants in the IEP meetings. However, the following are some points that should be taken into account in writing this part of the IEP:
>
> a. The statement should accurately describe the effect of the child's disability on the child's performance in any area of education that is affected, including:
>   1) academic areas (reading, math, communication, etc.), and
>   2) nonacademic areas (daily life activities, mobility, etc.)
>
> Appendix C of IDEA's regulations, 34 C.F.R. Part 300 (Response to Question No. 36)

As the previous excerpt indicates, special education includes both academic and nonacademic performance. Certainly occupational and physical therapists' expertise lies in assessing and treating the nonacademic components of performance. However, in a school setting, it is equally important for therapists to look at how a student's disability interferes with academic tasks. The challenge for therapists is to *translate* how a student's abilities and delays affect functional performance in school activities, ranging from physical education, art, and music to reading and writing. The first step is to identify a student's ability/disability profile and then explain how any delays affect performance. Therapists should use language that teachers and family members can easily understand.

Sarah is a third-grade student with traumatic brain injury resulting in a motor planning deficit (apraxia). Identifying that Sarah has motor planning problems is only one part of a therapist's responsibility to provide educationally relevant service. The impact of Sarah's motor deficit on her school performance must also be explained in simple terms; that is, Sarah's problems with sequencing and planning movements with her hands affects her ability to string cursive letters together smoothly across her paper when writing. As a result, she frequently stops and starts words and erases letters, creating messy papers as she struggles to keep up with the rest of the class.

In addition, all recommendations for intervention, whether for direct service or classroom consultation, must also be educationally relevant. This means that intervention must directly address the academic and nonacademic areas in which Sarah is not meeting the expectations of her educational team. Looking at Sarah's motor planning or gross and fine motor skills in isolation of her school performance is not educationally relevant. Certainly handwriting is one concern. Depending on Sarah's age, how she eats, puts on a coat, or plays on the swings and slide outside the classroom may be other important nonacademic areas possibly affected by poor motor planning. If Sarah were in tenth grade, these nonacademic areas would probably not be of concern to her teachers, but opening and closing her locker as well as navigating the hallways to reach each of her eight daily classes would be.

Criteria for Meeting Educational Relevance

Educational relevance is determined by the learning needs of each student, depending on age, grade in school, and ability. As described by one federal administrator of special education programs:

> In sum, the pertinent inquiry to be made in determining the extent of a school district's obligation to provide physical and occupational therapy is whether the child needs the services in order to benefit from special education. Please keep in mind that such an inquiry is dependent on the facts and circumstances of a particular case and therefore must be made on a case-by-case basis.
>
> Will 1988

The following four guidelines can help you determine whether or not your services are educationally relevant. Every school-based therapist should:

1. Identify *how* specific therapeutic domains (for example, sensory processing, neuromuscular functions, motor perception, and adaptive behavior) contribute to and/or challenge a student's performance in school.
2. Assess and describe a *student's performance* in specific areas of the school, such as the classroom, lunchroom, halls, playground, art class, and gymnasium, rather than solely on the basis of formal test results.
3. Discuss how intervention will *improve* the student's performance in academic subjects and other school activities.
4. Communicate, both verbally and through written reports, in *jargon-free language* that all team members can understand.

It is important to keep in mind that providing therapy in the classroom does not necessarily make it educationally relevant, *unless* the therapist's goals and activities are directed toward helping the student achieve the educational objectives agreed upon by the entire team, including family members. We have observed therapists who set up a therapy area in the classroom and bring in balls and mats to work individually with each student. These therapists claim they are providing school therapy, but they are actually setting up a clinic space in the classroom. In the same respect, giving teachers activities to implement in the classroom does not automatically make them educationally relevant, unless they also promote achievement of the student's educational outcomes. All therapeutic interventions, no matter who carries them out, must be related to the student's educational plan.

Therapeutic Domains and Educational Relevance

Occupational and physical therapists typically bring special expertise in five therapeutic domains to the educational setting:

- sensory awareness/processing
- neuromuscular functions
- motor (gross, fine, and oral-motor) skills
- perceptual skills
- adaptive behavior

While there may be some controversy about how to define areas of specialization and overlap between occupational and physical therapy, we have chosen not to distinguish between the two disciplines for our discussion of consultation in the schools and leave it up to the reader to decide who is prepared to address each of the five domains. Obviously, many of the domains overlap and students typically have problems in more than one domain at a time. Our list of therapeutic domains is not inclusive, since there are others that affect school performance; however, this categorization provides a systematic way to describe the educational outcomes, or relevance, of therapists' expertise in the schools. Rather than trying to improve a student's skills in these traditional domains, therapists must explain how they affect students' school performance and recommend intervention to help students achieve specific outcomes in academic and nonacademic areas.

Andy, a junior high school student with osteogenesis imperfecta, or brittle bones, has severe limitation of all movement and uses a wheelchair at school and at home. Andy and his teachers would like for him to work on his assignments independently in the classroom. Intervention to improve Andy's shoulder range of motion is a medical goal when viewed in isolation of how reduced movement in the shoulder affects his school performance. However, his consulting therapist, Ryan, addresses the educational relevance of this medical problem by explaining to Andy's teachers that he is unable to reach his books, paper, or pencil because of restricted shoulder movement. Ryan recommends that Andy's school materials be placed in a supply box attached to the side of his desk and demonstrates how to incorporate warm-up exercises and reaching activities within daily classroom routines to maintain the movement that Andy currently has. Ryan also shows Andy and his parents and teachers which movements to avoid since they will stress his joints. Particular emphasis is placed on consulting with Andy's physical education teacher.

The following sections describe the educational relevance of typical therapeutic domains addressed by therapists in the school setting and provide examples of consultation in the classroom, playground, and other school areas.

Sensory Awareness/Processing

Description

Sensory awareness/processing includes orienting to, receiving, differentiating, and interpreting somatosensory, vestibular, proprioceptive, visual, auditory, gustatory, and olfactory stimuli received from the environment and one's own body. Table 2.1 provides a summary of some desired educational outcomes and indicators of problems in sensory awareness/processing that are most likely to be observed in a school setting.

Table 2.1
Sensory Awareness/Processing and Relationship to School Performance

Subdomain	Educational Outcome	Indicators of Problems (Hyper- and Hyporeactive)
Somatosensory sensations include light touch, pressure, pain, and temperature	Identifies object or place on own body where sensation is received; discriminates between hugs, taps, tickles, and pinches during play and interaction with peers/adults; discriminates between hot and cold water, foods, and heat sources within classroom; uses classroom tools (pencils, pens, scissors) skillfully	Aversion to light touch, reacts by withdrawing from group activities or striking out at others; unresponsive to touch or does not know where body is touched
Vestibular and proprioception information includes changes in head/body position and direction and speed of movement	Exhibits fluid movements and changes in body position; coordinates eye movements for reading and copying from the board; understands how head and body are positioned	Avoids or craves movement, jogging, or rough play; has poor body scheme; has poor balance; maintains rigid posture or slumps in seat; exhibits mechanical motor performance

Table 2.1 (continued)

Subdomain	Educational Outcome	Indicators of Problems (Hyper- and Hyporeactive)
Visual information includes color, contrast, size, shape, and texture	Sees meaning by responding to color, shape, size, and contrast of symbols on a printed page, school supplies, furniture, peers' and teacher's clothing, and facial expressions	Does not notice details; cannot find materials; cannot focus on page, blackboard, or worksheet; seeks dim light
Auditory information includes rhythm, intonation, and intensity of sounds and speech	Uses understandable speech patterns; responds appropriately to sounds and direction (for example, lines up quickly when fire alarm rings or puts homework in specified box)	Dislikes loud and unexpected sounds (for example, fire bell or whistle); is distracted by or oblivious to background sounds and speech (such as ambulance in distance, student playing outside classroom, teacher writing on chalkboard)
Gustatory and olfactory information includes bitter, salty, sweet and sour tastes; scents and odors	Notices and responds appropriately to tastes and scents encountered daily in school (such as art materials, friend's lunch, classroom pets, janitor's cleaning materials, chalk dust); uses scents to recognize people and places	Eats same lunch every day or craves certain foods; explores environment by smelling everything or finds most scents offensive; has poor sucking, chewing, and swallowing skills

Examples of Educationally Relevant Consultation

Once a problem has been identified in a specific sensory system, school-based therapists must describe how the sensory information facilitates or impedes a student's school performance. For example, in addition to reporting that a student has a problem processing tactile and proprioceptive information, the impact of this deficit on school performance, particularly in relation to areas of concern defined by team members, must be explained. The following scenarios show how you might do so.

Chuck is an eight-year-old student with pervasive developmental delay. His teachers report that he is always sharpening pencils down to stubs, drumming the top of his desk, and pulling lint off his clothes. After identifying a sensory processing disorder, his therapist, Juan, explains that Chuck is attempting to increase the feedback he receives from his muscles, joints, and skin through pounding and pinching actions with his hands and arms. These actions provide important information about his body, which he does not receive when he sits still, and may help him remain alert. Juan and his team focused on ways to blend behavior management and sensory integrative approaches for interacting with Chuck. Juan recommended reinforcers for modifying Chuck's behavior, which would give him the type of sensory input he sought and appeared to enjoy so much. Sensorimotor activities that could be performed in the classroom, such as digging pennies out of soft clay balls or using a vibrating pen to make designs, were included in Chuck's daily schedule.

Asheesh, a preschool student with delayed language development, is highly distractible. Brad, his therapist, identifies that Asheesh has sensory defensiveness, a type of sensory integration disorder characterized by aversive responses to light touch and other sensory stimuli. He explains, "Asheesh is distracted by the students bumping up against his chair on their way to the water fountain because he is unusually sensitive to light touch. This is called sensory defensiveness. It would be helpful to move his desk to a quieter corner of the room. I also noticed that he seemed particularly distractible during his language group. I would like to talk with the speech-language pathologist to help her look out for other situations when he may be overstimulated by being touched lightly and unexpectedly."

Jake, a second-grade student with learning disabilities, was referred to Li, the school therapist, due to his extreme clumsiness and problems getting along with peers, which was particularly noticeable during PE and recess. Li observed that Jake was afraid to climb the slide or jungle gym and avoided bending over to pick up his pencil off the floor in the classroom. Further assessment pinpointed that gravitational insecurity, a sensory processing disorder involving the vestibular (movement and balance) system, was a major factor influencing Jake's behavior on the playground. Li offered an educationally relevant explanation for Jake's social isolation; that is, he feared climbing or getting into any position that tipped his head to the side or backward. She explained that his strategy for coping with his fear was to avoid fast-paced play and to keep his body firmly "planted" on the ground. Her recommendations included a combination of intensive direct service twice per week with reassessment at the end of three months and consultation with Jake's physical education and classroom teachers on a bi-monthly basis to find ways for Jake to participate comfortably in games with peers at recess and gym.

Neuromuscular Functions

Description

Therapists typically focus on the following components of nervous and musculoskeletal system functioning: muscle tone, range of motion of body joints, postural control, and body strength and endurance. These components are usually assessed through clinical observation and handling the student at rest and in motion. Table 2.2 provides a summary of some desired educational outcomes and indicators of problems in neuromuscular functions that are typically observed in a school setting.

Examples of Educationally Relevant Consultation

Therapists must look at how neuromuscular components affect a student's ability to assume and maintain the postures and positions needed to participate in daily school lessons and activities, including sports, physical education, science projects, handwriting, art, and lunch. An upright posture is critical for using hands and eyes in an efficient manner to manipulate school equipment, supplies, tools, and utensils. When students cannot assume and maintain upright postures themselves, therapists must advise educational staff regarding the choice and use of adapted seating and mobility options. Examples include recommending a slantboard for students with low muscle tone and poor wrist stability during writing periods or positioning

Table 2.2
Neuromuscular Functions and Relationship to School Performance

Components	Educational Outcome	Indicators of Problems
Muscle tone: degree of muscle tension or stiffness ***Range of motion:*** movement of body parts	Holds head, torso, and shoulders steady to move hands and eyes to attend and participate in classroom activities; moves body parts easily to reach school supplies, manipulate tools, and move throughout school environment	Muscles too loose or tight resulting in exaggerated or awkward movement, slumping in seat, propping head on hand or desk when writing or reading, sitting on feet or wrapping feet around chair legs; avoids fine motor tasks; writes as little as possible; movements are constricted; is messy with art projects
Postural control: ability to position self at rest and during activity	Sits upright comfortably to use hands and eyes for desktop work; stands to write at blackboard; carries lunch tray/books; positions self appropriately at play, sports, and recess	Has poor posture, especially when sitting and standing; exhibits problems holding steady while moving hands to write and color, or arms and legs to bat, kick, or shoot baskets
Strength and endurance: sustains self during exertion	Coordinates breathing and physical activity to maintain focus on task in classroom, play, or sports	Loses breath during activity; fatigues as day progresses

a student with severe neuromuscular involvement in a wheelchair with an abductor post, shoulder harness, and lap tray. Other positions, such as sidelying on the floor or lying prone on a wedge during circle time, are helpful for young children with significant physical disabilities.

Another classroom application of therapists' knowledge of the neuromuscular system is analyzing the energy requirements and developmental skills needed to perform specific school tasks. This information is critical for assisting educational staff to set priorities for tasks or know how long a student can engage in school activities before a break is required.

Mayra, a high school student with paraplegia following a bicycle accident when she was younger, is able to propel herself in her wheelchair around school, but doing so is exhausting and detracts from her ability to listen and take notes in class. While pushing her own wheelchair helps Mayra maintain her stamina, Yvonne, the consulting therapist, understands that this exertion takes too great a toll on her schoolwork. A plan is devised with Mayra to push herself until lunchtime; afterward friends will assist her to afternoon classes. Yvonne plans to reassess the situation in two months and encourages Mayra to join a wheelchair exercise class after school that is offered by the county recreation department.

Motor Skills

Description

Motor skills can be subdivided into three interrelated categories:

Gross motor skills include coordination and balance, bilateral integration (using both sides of the body in a coordinated manner), and praxis (motor planning).

Fine/visual motor skills include hand preference and separation of the hands for skill and power, manipulation (patterns of grasp and release, development of hand arches and in-hand manipulation), visual-motor integration and crossing the midline of the body with hands and eyes.

Oral-motor skills include coordination of breathing, chewing, and swallowing; tongue, lip, and jaw posture and movement; oral reflexes; and movements of the tongue, lips, and cheeks for talking and eating.

Tables 2.3, 2.4, and 2.5 provide a summary of the desired educational outcomes and indicators of problems in gross, fine\visual motor, and oral-motor skills frequently observed in the school environment.

Table 2.3
Gross Motor Skills and Relationship to School Performance

Components	Educational Outcome	Indicators of Problems
Motor coordination and balance: Fluid movement as needed to successfully complete activity	Maintains and changes position easily in groups on the floor, in and out of chairs, and other school furniture and equipment; enjoys playground and physical education activities	Bumps into desks, walls, or other children; has poor ball skills; has problems stopping and starting precise movement in physical education
Bilateral integration: Uses both sides of the body simultaneously and reciprocally during an activity	Climbs stairs, catches and throws ball, passes objects easily from hand to hand, pushes chair across room, understands left/right orientation	Loses balance on playground; goes up and down stairs two-footed (after 4 years of age); has difficulty pumping a swing, dribbling a ball, or clapping rhythms; confuses left and right
Motor planning: thinking of and planning a new motor act	Knows how to move body as needed during games and classroom activities; follows directions easily, especially when new or multiple actions are involved (for example, uses a compass in math)	Appears clumsy in sports and games; resists changing routines; avoids new activities or takes a long time to learn them; labors over handwriting

Table 2.4
Fine/Visual Motor Skills and Relationship to School Performance

Components	Educational Outcome	Indicators of Problems
Hand preference: using one hand for skilled tasks and the other to assist	Uses one hand to manipulate tools for coloring, writing, eating, pasting, cutting, and other tasks while other hand holds object; works comfortably with body/hands at center of work space	Has not established lead and assist hands; uses either hand ineffectively for tasks such as writing, eating, and cutting; has problems zipping, buttoning, cutting, and using stencils or templates
Manipulation: holding and handling small objects with power and skill	Opens milk carton or jar; holds pencil, pen, crayon, brush in mature grasp to color, write, and draw; turns pencil over with lead hand to use eraser; cuts with scissors; is successful with art projects; zips, buttons, and ties clothing; manipulates puzzles; uses counting blocks in math; turns pages of books	Immature grip; hand shakes when writing; is clumsy with writing tools and art supplies, buttons, and zippers; breaks toys/materials; glues and cuts with difficulty; bends pages when turning them; uses two hands to erase or change pencil grasp
Visual-motor integration: coordination of visual information with action	Guides hands visually for skilled movement, cuts on lines, colors within boundaries, catches ball, threads needle	Avoids art tasks and play with blocks; colors outside boundaries; cuts off lines with scissors, especially curves
Crossing the midline: using each hand on either side of the body as needed	Is comfortable using hands to reach for, retrieve, and grasp materials placed on desktops, on tables, in cupboards, and on other surfaces	Uses left hand in left work space and right hand in right work space; ignores part of work space; switches chalk/pencil to other hand when writing/drawing, especially big letters or pictures

Table 2.5
Oral-Motor Skills and Relationship to School Performance

Components	Educational Outcome	Indicators of Problems
Oral-motor skills: Coordination of sucking, swallowing, biting, chewing, blowing, breathing, and speaking	Eats independently and neatly, speaks clearly, plays woodwind instruments in band, blows whistle	Drools, eats messily (mouth open, does not chew food thoroughly), demonstrates primitive reflexes such as tongue thrust, poor articulation of speech sounds

Examples of Educationally Relevant Consultation

Gross Motor Skills

Gross motor skills affect how students coordinate their body positions and move fluidly from one location to another within the classroom and other school environments as well as participate in physical education, play, and sports activities.

Sheila, a seven-year-old girl with juvenile rheumatoid arthritis, has gross motor skills at the four-year-old level and has particular problems with balance, endurance, and speed of movement. Lynn, her therapist, addresses educational relevance by identifying Sheila's motor abilities and delays as well as describing their impact on her performance in school. She explains, "Sheila's stiffness and limited motion in her joints makes it difficult for her to get in and out of her seat and finish class assignments in the allotted time."

Lynn explores other school-related issues with Sheila's teacher. She discusses the best kind of seating for Sheila, the height of her desk and chair, and accessibility of school supplies. Lynn recommends that Sheila use an electric pencil sharpener at her desk to eliminate an extra trip out of her seat as well as protect her wrists from pushing too hard in an awkward position with the manual pencil sharpener. Lynn shows Sheila, her teacher, and the classroom assistants the safest ways for her to use the playground equipment. She also consults with Sheila's physical education teacher to plan how she can participate with her class during PE.

Fine/Visual Motor Skills

Fine motor skills affect how students use their eyes and hands to handle objects as well as communicate manually through gestures or sign language. Educationally relevant practice addresses how problems in this domain affect students' abilities to manipulate classroom tools such as rulers, compasses, pencils, erasers, crayons, paintbrushes, chalk, and scissors. Fine/visual motor skills enable students to take care of personal needs, such as zipping and buttoning clothing, securing a bathroom lock, holding a spoon or fork, opening milk cartons, unwrapping lunch, and turning the pages of a book.

Writing is one of the primary educational outcomes of the fine/visual motor domain. Lack of fine/visual motor skill is a major reason why a student may have difficulty with manual communication, which includes putting thoughts and ideas on paper, typing on a typewriter or computer, or using sign language. Computer literacy is part of the educational curriculum in many schools today and fine/visual motor skills are crucial for using a keyboard. If students experience difficulty using computers, changes in body position and equipment adaptations can facilitate the development of these skills. Some students have very limited fine/visual motor abilities; rather than trying to develop children's wrist stability and finger extension, the therapist could consult with the educational team to develop an alternative plan, such as substituting a head stick to depress keys or using a joystick and scanning program to light up the alphabet letter by letter.

Coloring, drawing, and painting are also forms of manual self-expression that are dependent upon fine/visual motor skills. Completing art projects; using a stapler, paper clips, scotch tape, and glue; and participating in vocational education classes such as wood shop are important school skills.

One very bright second-grade boy, Andy, avoided all forms of written expression, including coloring and drawing. Shula, his school therapist, observed Andy during language arts and watched him illustrate his story with his right hand while his left hand remained in his lap. Frustrated that the paper was moving too much, Andy looked around the room for a self-stick note to secure his paper instead of using his left hand to hold it. Shula determined that Andy did not use a lead and assist hand because of poor bilateral integration. She met with Andy's teacher and parents and described how his inability to use both sides of the body together in a coordinated manner detracted from using a lead and helper hand so necessary for skill in writing or drawing. Recommending a combination of direct service and classroom consultation, Shula and the teacher developed a plan to verify which hand to encourage Andy to use as the lead and determined how to simplify the motor demands of other classroom tasks, such as cutting with small scissors and using heavier construction paper so it would not flop over Andy's hands as he cut.

Oral-Motor Skills

In the school environment, the two primary outcomes of oral-motor development are eating/drinking and the production of sounds for speech. The tongue, lip, and cheek muscles produce sucking, chewing, and swallowing movements for eating as well as help produce sounds for speech. Most students eat lunch at school and often have snacks during breaks or special celebrations.

Jana is a four-year-old preschooler with cerebral palsy who has significant oral-motor reflexes. The impact of her tongue thrust and bite reflex must be described in understandable terms to Nina, the classroom assistant who feeds Jana every day. Julian, the school therapist, explains, "When Jana bites down hard on the spoon she is demonstrating a reflex, an action she cannot control. Tugging the spoon out of her mouth and scraping her lips and chin after each mouthful only triggers her reflexes." An individualized feeding program for Jana was developed by Julian in consultation with Nina and Jana's mother. They decided that Julian would come twice a week for two weeks to demonstrate how to hold Jana and offer her food. Afterward, Julian consulted with Jana and Nina once per week at lunch time to monitor progress and make adjustments as needed. Jana's mother joined their sessions at school twice per month so she could feed Jana the same way at home. Julian also consulted with Jana's speech-language pathologist once per month to demonstrate proper positioning during language activities in the classroom. At the same time, Julian learned which sounds to encourage when he saw Jana each week.

Perceptual Skills

Description

This domain represents a collection of skills that support learning and are based on the ability to organize sensory information from the environment and one's body into meaningful patterns to develop:

- attention
- visual perceptual functions, such as form constancy, position in space, visual closure, figure ground discrimination, spatial relationships, and depth perception
- body scheme, including left/right orientation
- orientation to time, place, and situation
- spatial awareness.

Table 2.6 provides a summary of some desired educational outcomes and indicators of perceptual skills problems that are most frequently observed in the school environment.

Table 2.6
Perceptual Skills and Relationship to School Performance

Components	Educational Outcome	Indicators of Problems
Attention: state of arousal and alertness for school activities	Focuses on task at hand despite competing sounds, sights, actions, and touch; maintains appropriate attention for activity (quiet or active)	Is inattentive, loses attention frequently; has difficulty refocusing once distracted; may also be very tense and overly focused on one aspect of a task
Visual perception: recognition of shape, color, size, and position in space	Recognizes and finds class supplies, recognizes letters for reading, draws or writes letters/shapes, organizes worksheets and lessons, as well as columns and numbers in math	Has difficulty matching colors and shapes and copying letters, loses place on page, reverses words in reading/writing, rotates paper when drawing/writing, does not recognize written errors, needs a model for writing, is inconsistent or has poor slant when writing, cannot do construction projects
Body scheme: internal awareness of body and all its parts	Understands how to move body parts without watching to eat, play, write, and engage in other activities; moves fluidly in school; draws complete person (5+ years old)	Draws human figure lacking critical parts (inappropriate for age); loses hats, gloves, and coat; watches hands and feet when learning new task
Orientation to time and place: knows what is happening and has sense of time	Understands layout of the classroom and school, knows where to find supplies and materials, understands daily schedule	Puts belongings/materials in wrong places, cannot find needed materials, forgets schedule, appears confused or frustrated
Spatial awareness: understands relationship of objects to one another and to self	Completes puzzles, builds with blocks, writes within lines/margins, participates in team sports and PE	Has problems building from block patterns/models; runs in wrong direction, misjudges distance or where ball will land in PE; loses direction around school

Examples of Educationally Relevant Consultation

Perceptual skills are very familiar to educators but not necessarily to family members. For students functioning at the preschool and kindergarten level, the development of perceptual skills is generally considered a major part of the curriculum as children work on recognizing shapes and letters, focus on details in a picture, form a mental image of the human figure and draw it, and understand the position of objects to one another and to oneself in order to comprehend prepositions such as *under, over,* and *behind.* For older students, problems in this domain will detract from their performance in sports, higher-level math (geometry), and general problem-solving skills needed to organize notes, write reports, and make class presentations. All students, no matter what their age, must have the appropriate orienting and attending skills to learn when to listen and focus on classroom activities and when they can "goof off."

Visual perception is a critical skill for learning to read and write. Students must perceive the shape, size, and form of letters and numbers so that they can learn the appropriate sound-symbol association necessary for reading. Students also learn to recall and produce the shape and form of letters and numbers to space letters, words, sentences, or drawings on a page.

Orientation to time and space is another skill necessary for remembering how to find the lunchroom or gymnasium, tell what day or season it is, know where school supplies are kept, and understand when assignments are due. Daily routines in many early childhood classes begin with identifying the day of the week, date, weather conditions, and a description of daily news events. Older students have homerooms at the beginning and end of the day and are expected to remember and meet class routines and follow rules and schedules. Table 2.7 shows the common activities that students encounter in a typical school day. Note how many of these typical activities are nonacademic. Knowing students' class schedules will enable therapists to provide services that complement and do not disrupt established routines. Field trips, community service, and vocational education internships are part of most school programs and provide important opportunities for consulting therapists to observe and modify student behavior and performance in environments outside the school setting.

Darnel, a ten-year-old student with severe learning disabilities, has just joined a regular fifth-grade classroom after two years in a self-contained LD class. His therapist, Aaron, is consulting with Darnel's teachers to help them understand and adjust to his visual perception problems. In math, students sit four to a table rather than at individual desks to work on math "teasers" together. Darnel's group was usually the last to finish because they bickered about sharing materials. From the teacher's viewpoint, Darnel could not cooperate to resolve a problem. After observing Darnel in the classroom, Aaron pointed out how Darnel's perceptual problems interfered with his ability to keep his belongings and supplies organized; that is, without the boundary of his desk top, Darnel was mixing his blocks and supplies with those of the other students. Since he was not able to keep track of his math supplies on his own, Aaron suggested that the students put each of their forms on a different colored paper and use white sheets for their common work.

Table 2.7
Typical School Activities and Routines
(Note: nonacademic items are in italics)

Transportation/Mobility		Instructional Time	
travel to and from school by walking, car, or bus		language	reading/writing
getting around classroom/school		visual perception	math
		self-help skills	social studies
		socialization	science
		fine and gross motor	
Opening and Closing Routines		**Specials**	
putting coats and materials in cubbie/locker homeroom		*art*	*physical education*
morning and closing announcements/pledge		*music/drama*	*field trips*
calendar/weather/review of daily schedule		library	*vocational education*
		assemblies	
Class Jobs/Responsibilities		**Other**	
office messenger	*line leader*	*lunch and snack*	*extracurricular activities*
hand out supplies	*safety patrol*	*recess and free time*	study hall
hall monitor	*peer tutor*		
student council	*community service*		

Adaptive Behavior

Description

The focus of this domain is on the skills needed to fulfill student roles and responsibilities in the schools, including social interaction and conduct, problem-solving and coping behavior, and self-control. While it may appear to some therapists that this is not one of the standard domains for which they provide services, we urge both physical and occupational therapists to pay particular attention to the impact of sensory processing, perceptual, neuromuscular, and motor concerns on the development of psychosocial skills, as illustrated in Luke's vignette at the end of this section. Table 2.8 provides a summary of some desired educational outcomes and indicators of problems with adaptive behavior that are typically observed in a school environment.

Examples of Educationally Relevant Consultation

In the school environment, a child's major social roles are that of student and friend; by the age of 16 years, the role of community worker also assumes a major role as students prepare to leave school and continue their education or enter the work force.

Table 2.8
Adaptive Behavior and Relationship to School Performance

Components	Educational Outcome	Indicators of Problems
Social interaction: relating positively to peers and adults	Demonstrates behavior appropriate to the situation; participates in team games, sports, and other extracurricular activities; plays/works cooperatively with others	Does not know how to make friends, join groups, initiate and maintain conversation; does not follow class rules, take turns, or share materials
Social problem solving: setting up appropriate goals and choosing task-specific strategies	Knows when to ask for help; manages time well; has good problem-solving skills; handles disputes with peers; knows when to work and when to play	Dawdles, forgets directions and routines, withdraws or acts out during group times, seeks adult intervention inappropriately to resolve problems with others, jokes at inappropriate times
Self-control: regulating and adjusting own responses	Recognizes own feelings and those of others and acts accordingly, responds appropriately to verbal and nonverbal cues	Exhibits eye contact and intensity of voice inappropriate for situation, interrupts conversations, ignores personal space of others, is easily overstimulated and unfocused

In the course of daily school activities, students need to discriminate among how to interact with friends versus teachers, resolve disagreements in sports and play, express emotions and needs appropriately, manage time to complete assignments, accept limits, and meet their own and teachers' expectations regarding classroom assignments. Many elementary school teachers rotate classroom "chores" among class members, such as delivering lunch money and attendance sheets to the office, being at the head of the line, and collecting work or handing out paper for written assignments. Junior and senior high school students participate in social activities such as extracurricular clubs related to leisure or future career interests, school councils, and vocational education classes where they learn specific job-related skills as well as critical work attitudes and values.

All students, no matter what their age, must be able to sequence ideas, plan their actions, know when to ask for help, and work cooperatively with others, including fellow students, teachers, and job placement supervisors. Difficulty with social problem solving will interfere with school behaviors, such as figuring out how to correct a mistake; seeking help; following directions; and organizing supplies, homework, backpacks, lockers, and desks.

Obviously, problems in any of the domains previously discussed will affect an individual's social and adaptive behavior in school. By providing explanations for how problems in their areas of expertise affect behavior, therapists can suggest alternative ways for the educational team to assist students to participate in age-appropriate activities during the school day. In addition, therapists can look for opportunities to promote students' adaptive behavior; for example, including classmates in intervention and focusing on performance during group and social activities in school can provide opportunities to improve relationship skills.

Think again about Chuck, the student with pervasive developmental delay introduced in the section on sensory processing in this chapter. In addition to helping Chuck's teachers use enjoyable reinforcers, Juan provided integrated therapy in Chuck's classroom one morning per week. For example, Juan introduced a vibrating pen to Chuck for making designs and a squirt bottle filled with water for identifying laminated letters spread out on a cafeteria tray (instead of pointing with his finger). The vibrations from the pen as well as pumping the squirt bottle provided the kind of sensations that calmed Chuck while he completed equally important class lessons. In addition, Juan incorporated another of Chuck's goals, to improve peer interaction, by setting up the letter recognition activity so he could take turns with a classmate to squirt the bottle.

Luke, a fifth-grade student with emotional problems, had difficulty getting along in group games and frequently stomped away in tears, believing that the other children were not playing fairly. After observing his behavior on the playground, Mary, the school therapist, noticed that Luke behaved much better when playing board games or simple action games, such as tag. With further assessment, she found that Luke had many balance and motor problems, especially with sequencing the fast-paced action that occurred during kickball and other sports. When a ball was kicked his way, Luke's classmates would all shout simultaneously what to do, further confusing him. He needed time to process how to catch the ball before figuring out which base to throw it to. Consulting with Luke's teacher led to the development of a stop-gap plan: Luke would play catcher and concentrate on returning the ball to one person, the pitcher. The longer-term plan involved ways to help Luke learn to cope with his frustrations before walking out of the game and to improve his running, particularly around corners or when running the bases. The other students were also encouraged to rotate the role of "coach" among themselves so that only one person at a time would give directions to Luke.

Conclusion

The effective use of consultation in schools is dependent upon identifying the educational relevance of common therapeutic domains. In order to improve student performance, consulting therapists must use their expertise and knowledge to assist others to fulfill their roles. This means helping family members, teachers, and other specialists to incorporate specially designed intervention in meaningful ways throughout their daily interactions and instruction with students. The primary task is to facilitate a goodness-of-fit for students in their educational placements, whether the setting is a community preschool, regular or special education classroom, school lunchroom, or vocational education site.

In order to plan educationally relevant consultation, therapists must critically analyze three interrelated components of the consulting situation:

Student's profile of abilities, functional problems, and educational outcomes. It is important to analyze the abilities that a student has and uses to enhance school performance, as well as where the barriers to learning in academic and nonacademic areas lie. This analysis will lead to the identification of educational outcomes to guide recommendations for intervention.

Role and function of key human resources involved in promoting school performance. Consultation assists others who have frequent contact with the child, including family members and caregivers, special and general educators, classroom assistants, bus drivers, psychologists, speech-language pathologists, and social workers. One of the primary benefits of consultation is the enhancement of the unique knowledge and experiences of team members, as well as your own.

How the environment facilitates or deters the student's school performance. The primary school environment is the classroom. However, other areas of the school have an equally important impact on student performance and include specific learning areas within a classroom, such as the reading corner or gross motor area, lunchroom, bathroom, hallways, gymnasium, playground, art and music rooms, vocational education areas, and study halls.

Figure 2.1 illustrates the relationships among these key components. Each component is discussed in detail in the following three chapters.

Figure 2.1
Components of School-Based Consultation

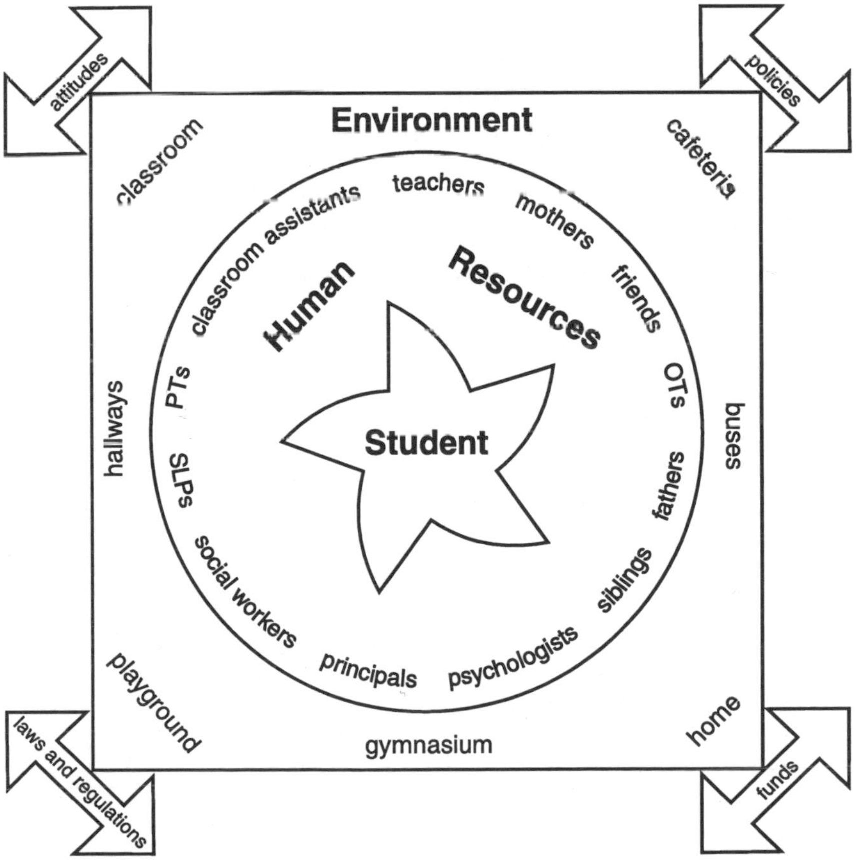

Selected Readings

Bundy, A., and R. Carter. 1991. *A conceptual model of practice for school system therapists.* Chicago: University of Illinois.

This instructional package of a model curriculum for school-based therapists includes videotaped case studies showing how to provide educationally relevant services. The videos show a first-grade boy with cerebral palsy included in a general classroom and a kindergartner with hyperactivity and learning disabilities in a self-contained classroom. The project was developed with federal funds by the Departments of Occupational and Physical Therapy at the University of Illinois at Chicago. (College of Associated Health Professions, 1919 W. Taylor Street, Chicago, Illinois 60612)

Effgen, S. 1994. The educational environment. In *Physical therapy for children,* edited by S. Campbell, R. Palisano, and D. Vanderlinden. Philadelphia: Saunders.

Based on a systems approach to school-based practice, the author offers guidelines for providing physical therapy services in an educational environment.

Giangreco, M., J. York, and B. Rainforth. 1989. Providing related services to learners with severe handicaps in the educational setting: Pursuing the least restrictive option. *Pediatric Physical Therapy* 55-63.

A continuum of therapy services is presented in this article that describes how therapy is related to educational programming through integrated intervention in school activities.

Golubock, S., and S. Reed. 1991. Meeting a student's needs by asking the right questions. In *School-based practice for related services, lesson 3,* edited by C. Royeen. Bethesda, MD: American Occupational Therapy Association.

Part of a self-study series about working in the schools, Lesson 3 focuses on a central tenet of educational relevance—how to ask the right questions to identify which services are needed to meet the needs of students with learning problems. The application to practice sections are individualized for occupational and physical therapy and speech-language pathology.

Niehaus, A., A. Bundy, C. Mattingly, and M. Lawlor. 1991. Making a difference: Occupational therapy in the public schools. *Occupational Therapy Journal of Research* 11(4):195-212.

This narrative study of the practice of five expert occupational therapists provides insight into the ways in which educationally relevant services were developed over time, particularly how the therapists reframed or explained student behavior with regard to the impact of their medical diagnoses on school performance.

Orelove, F., and D. Sobsey, Eds. 1991. *Educating children with multiple disabilities.* Baltimore: Paul H. Brookes.

This text emphasizes a collaborative team approach to working with students with multiple disabilities in the educational setting. It includes excellent chapters written by pediatric occupational and physical therapists on the sensorimotor system, handling and positioning students, and developing instructional adaptations for the classroom.

Rainforth, B., J. York, and C. MacDonald. 1992. *Collaborative teams for students with severe disabilities.* Baltimore: Paul H. Brookes.

This resource addresses the issue of educationally relevant services for students with severe disabilities. The authors, two physical therapists and a speech-language pathologist, describe a transdisciplinary model of integrated therapy in which therapists and other members of the education team design comprehensive programs for students in a variety of daily school situations. Integrated therapy combines direct and consultative service in the classroom and other school environments.

Royeen, C., Ed. 1992. *Classroom applications for school-based practice.* Rockville, MD: American Occupational Therapy Association.

This self-study series of nine lessons highlights occupational therapy intervention in the classroom. Lesson 1 discusses educationally relevant assessments and evaluations for occupational therapists and gives examples of procedures and documentation of results. Other topics address handwriting and hand function, reading and visual perception, communication and behavior, mobility and seating, adaptive equipment and technology, oral-motor/feeding issues, and transition planning and services.

Chapter 3 focuses on the first component of our school-based consulting model, the student's profile of abilities and functional problems. Chapter highlights include:

- guidelines for observing student performance during education tasks
- application of these guidelines through the observation of two students engaged in school activities and lessons—a fourth-grader with learning disabilities and a preschooler with autism

Chapter 3

Analyzing Student Performance in the School Environment

> *There are a lot of little things that a child has to do at school . . . hold onto a pencil, not break the lead, change from one task to another, recognize stop signs on the way to school . . . compete in sports . . . pay attention to a roomful of people . . . do things fast . . . or do them slowly . . . do two things at once . . .*
>
> Ayres 1979

School performance must be viewed as a process that changes over time. Any one observation is only a window of opportunity to view student behavior and performance during specific academic and nonacademic tasks, such as taking tests, completing worksheets, playing with friends, and moving around the classroom and through hallways. Uri Bronfenbrenner, a developmental psychologist, once described research in contemporary developmental psychology "as the science of the strange behavior of children in strange situations with strange adults for the briefest possible period of time" (Bronfenbrenner 1977). His statement stands as an important ideal for all therapists who observe students in school: look at performance in a functional, not isolated, context to see typical behavior. This chapter focuses attention on the behaviors that students need to be successful in school.

Observing Student Performance

When you first see a student and begin talking to key team members, the challenge you face as a consulting therapist is to determine how typical the child's behaviors and skills are and what their impact is on learning and interaction with peers and adults at school. Your observations, assessments, and discussions with team members should provide information about why the student is behaving in certain ways. These elements should also lead to recommendations for improving the student's performance.

The form Observing Student Performance in School (see figures 3.1 and 3.2, pages 45-48) is an observation guide organized by nine parameters of student performance that occupational and physical therapists would be likely to observe in a classroom or other school environment. (A blank form that you may reproduce for your own use is included in the appendix.) These parameters were chosen because they represent behaviors that are valued by educators and are readily observed in typical classroom activities without bringing in special therapy equipment or test protocols. Each parameter is discussed in the following sections. Case examples are interspersed to illustrate key points.

The observation guide is intended to focus your initial classroom observations on student performance and should not replace formal assessments. In the same respect, formal assessment cannot substitute for classroom/school observations of performance. Both are needed to clarify a student's behavior and ability profile in order to develop an intervention plan. Keep in mind that assessing a student's performance is only one of three components of the school-based consultation model. Two other critical parts of your consultation analysis should include the experience and knowledge of human resources (family members, other specialists, and your own), and the influence of the school environment on a student's performance. Suggestions in the selected reading list at the end of this chapter will provide you with resources for additional observation forms and procedures.

Purpose of the Task

Start your observation by understanding the educational activity that the student is engaged in during your observation. The subject or task could range from lessons in physical education, music, math, or language arts to lunchroom behavior or play during recess. Find out what the objective of the lesson or activity is so you can judge how the student's behavior and ability profile affect successful performance of the task under observation. If you are observing a student who already has an IEP, judge performance on the task in relation to progress toward attaining IEP goals and objectives.

Nature of the Activity

The student may be requested to work independently, with a partner, or in a small cooperative group. All three of these situations require different types of interaction, and consequently, different levels of skill and processing of information. Cooperative learning is a popular trend in education and involves small groups of students pooling their knowledge to solve a task, such as performing a science experiment together or reading a story, acting out the parts, and answering related questions.

Although any school activity you observe can be classified by subject area and learning objectives, a task analysis will reveal parts dependent on motor, perceptual, sensory processing, neuromuscular, and psychosocial abilities. As an OT or PT, you have expertise in these nonacademic therapeutic domains (see chapter 2). As you observe the student performing a school activity, look at each part of the task and analyze the domains involved. Use your therapeutic knowledge to explain why the student may not successfully complete all or part of the task. This analysis is the essence of educational relevance.

The observed task also involves one of three primary learning channels, hearing (auditory), seeing (visual), and doing (tactile, proprioception and vestibular), upon which the majority of all school activities depend. Your understanding of neuromuscular functions and sensory processing principles, for example, is the basis for analyzing how students take in, integrate, and use sensory information to learn in school. Auditory input comes from listening to a teacher or a peer, while visual input is provided by looking at what is written on the blackboard, book, or worksheet or watching a demonstration by the teacher or another student. Tactile, proprioceptive, and vestibular input includes touching materials/tools to hold a pencil, build with blocks, sculpt with clay, or manipulate Cuisenaire rods or a fork. These systems also provide the student with information about movement in physical education, body position while sitting in a chair, or navigation in the classroom aisles to walk to the pencil sharpener without stumbling and tripping. As a consulting therapist, your knowledge of how motor and sensory systems affect learning is a unique contribution to the school setting since most educators typically focus on listening and reading for learning.

Examples of Purpose of the Task and Nature of the Activity

Sharmane is a fourth-grade student in general education who was recently diagnosed with learning disabilities. When you arrive for your observation, she is completing a language arts worksheet on her own and is trying to answer seven questions about the story that her reading group has just finished reading aloud. Her performance on this visual-motor task gives you an opportunity to observe her fine motor skills when she writes, her posture as she holds her pencil, and her problem-solving skills if she cannot answer all the questions. You will also have an opportunity to observe her organizational skills and ability to work independently. Sharmane will use visual and tactile information to read the worksheet, place her letters on the appropriate lines, and grip the pencil appropriately. Vestibular and proprioceptive input influence her posture while she is seated at the desk and when she bends over to pick her pencil off the floor or rummages in her desk for another eraser. (Note that completing this worksheet is also dependent upon Sharmane's cognitive skills, since she must decode the written symbols, derive meaning from them to understand the directions, remember the story, compose answers to the worksheet questions in her mind, and then write legibly in cursive using correct capitalization, punctuation, and grammar. These skills tap the expertise of her teachers, including her classroom teacher and probably a special educator, rather than an occupational or physical therapist.)

In another example, Nathan, a five-year-old boy with autism, is hyperactive, with reportedly poor motor skills and balance. You have been asked to observe Nathan in adaptive physical education with the rest of his class of eight students to develop an intervention plan with his teacher, Mr. G. His IEP goals and objectives include the following for motor development: will track and catch a 10" inflatable ball to participate in adaptive PE games/activities and will use two hands to carry a lunch tray with sandwich and milk carton 10 feet in the school cafeteria. Mr. G. has set up four stations in the gymnasium for the students to rotate through in pairs. Each station has a perceptual-motor activity involving throwing, passing, kicking, or running with an inflatable ball. Nathan's performance on these perceptual-motor paired tasks gives you an opportunity to view his gross motor skills and watch his response to fast-paced movement. He seeks out heavy touch pressure and pounding by kicking the ball over and over and throwing himself on a pile of mats off to the side. The high ceilings create echos as the students shout, which appear to distract Nathan. Even though four centers are set up, their boundaries are unmarked and there is no clear path from one to the other. You will see how Nathan responds to this lack of structure. (The appendix includes a form for evaluating the impact of the school environment on student performance; an example is completed in figure 3.2 for Nathan during his adaptive PE class.)

Accuracy of Performance

This parameter focuses on how the student approaches and completes a task, not just whether the task is finished on time. Which parts of the task are completed successfully? Which parts are difficult? It is as important to look at what the student is capable of doing as where the difficulty lies. When problems are encountered, does the student compensate or try to adapt? How is the problem solved; for example, by looking for visual clues, asking questions, or trial and error? Perhaps during a problem-solving situation the student becomes inattentive—an important observation since the student may really be frustrated by the demands of a task and not truly distractible.

Examples of Accuracy of Performance

Sharmane finishes only three questions on her worksheet while the other children in her group complete the entire worksheet. Why? You observed her sharpen her pencil twice before looking at the worksheet, giggle with the girl sitting next to her, and then hunt around in her desk for her reading book before she began. By this time the other students were on questions 3 and 4. When she finally began writing, she started on question 2, wrote two words, erased both several times, started over, and looked to see what her neighbor had written. You also observed that when Sharmane held her pencil, she used an immature grip and pressed very hard on the pencil, creating a dark, heavy line that was hard to erase and write over neatly. Her feet were planted firmly on the floor but the desk was too low, causing Sharmane to bend her neck and lean over her worksheet.

From this observation, you have formulated several questions in your mind. Is this typical behavior? You think so because one of the teacher's complaints is that Sharmane takes too long to complete her assignments. Is Sharmane avoiding writing because it is difficult for her? What are her visual-perceptual and fine motor abilities? There could also be a language deficit related to information retrieval or even reading comprehension, but these factors are beyond the expertise of an occupational or physical therapist to analyze. Still, it would be helpful to know if they have been checked out. You also wonder about her organizational skills and want to check out her ability to sequence her actions. Again, a language or cognitive assessment would give you information on her ability to sequence and verbalize her thoughts. Perhaps she can tell you her answers much better than she can write them, or she may not be able to do either.

After watching Mr. G. demonstrate what to do at each of the four stations in PE, Nathan runs wildly to the first center, grabs the ball, and kicks it away. He laughs and shouts as he runs after the ball and keeps kicking it around the gymnasium. You make several immediate observations about his performance. He doesn't seem to be able to listen and follow directions, even simple ones with a demonstration. Balls excite him and unstructured running quickly escalates his hyperactive behavior. However, you're pleasantly surprised by his ability to drop-kick the ball accurately against the wall and his ability to veer away from running into another student or piece of equipment at the last second. His running is smooth, with good weight shifts. In addition, his ability to stand on one foot for the drop-kick indicates age-appropriate balance skills.

You wonder what happens to Nathan's balance if he slows down. Is he dependent on movement and pounding input to his legs to activate his balance? Mr. G. has already told you that Nathan has problems with balance; he cannot carry his lunch tray in the cafeteria or materials around the classroom without bumping into things. Maybe what the teacher is observing is more a problem with sequencing movement or visualizing space than a balance problem. You will need to investigate further.

Attention to Activity

The Attention to Activity section relates to how well the student focuses on each part of the task you observe. If the student is distracted, what was the nature of the distraction? Was it a sight, sound, or action? In particular, what sensations were part of the distraction; for instance, was the child touched or moved? Were sounds loud and sudden, causing the student to clap both hands over the ears? Or was there no particular sensory event that triggered the distraction? One other important observation relates to how easily the student can refocus attention on the task at hand once disrupted. Is a physical prompt, such as firm touch, helpful or are verbal directions sufficient?

Handling Transitions

This parameter is closely related to attention but focuses on a student's independence in the school setting, as well as organizational abilities. As a physical or occupational therapist, you are particularly interested in how students' sensory, perceptual, motor, and interpersonal abilities aid them in changing their focus to work on different tasks throughout the day. The ability to sequence and plan movement is an important part of the transition from one task to another, such as coming in to homeroom, taking off coat and hat, and settling down to begin the first lesson or activity of the day. Students must also make transitions between areas of the school; for instance, when changing classes, going to lunch, or going on a field trip.

During your observation, look at what happens when the student completes the task or when time runs out. Does the student know what to do next? How much instruction or direction is needed to end the task and transition to another? Are there specific routines to follow for cleanup or for uncompleted work? Does the student appear to understand what is expected? Can the student move on and begin the next task, even if moving to another area of the classroom or school is required? How do previous activities influence the student's performance and what elements carry over to the new task? For example, did the class just return from lunch where they had a chance to move around or are they beginning another lesson that requires paying attention and sitting still?

Examples of Attention to Activity and Handling Transitions

As you have noted from previous examples, Sharmane had problems getting started on her task. Perhaps she did not have a clear idea of what she needed to do or what the parts of the task were. You observe that when she gets lost, she looks to her neighbor to see what to do. Visual input, in the form of a model, is helpful to Sharmane and she appears to be able to translate what she sees into action. This is positive information to investigate further and share with Sharmane's teacher, who appears frustrated that Sharmane is not completing her work, even when given explicit instructions. It may be that auditory information is not as helpful as visual information for Sharmane. Perhaps an assessment of her auditory processing should be recommended.

Nathan definitely has problems with paying attention and handling transitions. You have noticed that the walk through the halls to PE class has overstimulated him and the fast-paced action during PE class increases his distractibility. Does this happen frequently when Nathan changes activities or locations? If so, some calming techniques might be helpful before starting a new task. The big question to answer is, what type of input would be calming for Nathan? Once overstimulated, he does not respond to verbal directions or modeling.

Problem Solving

Problem solving is a complex set of behaviors that enable a student to develop an appropriate option for resolving daily academic, social, and personal dilemmas associated with successful school performance. Such dilemmas include figuring out how to put your pencil in the new sharpener, telling a friend to return a special eraser, letting the teacher know you have the right answer, and getting yourself positioned correctly to go down a slide. Observe to see whether the student understands and follows directions, has a plan of what to do, and makes changes to the plan if a problem arises.

Organization

Following class routines and organizing work space and schedules are important components of successful student behavior. Pay special attention to the student's organization of three-dimensional space, including desk, cubby, and backpack. Does the student find needed materials right away or pull everything out during the search for the right items? Some schools no longer use separate desks for each student and instead organize small cooperative learning groups at a table. Observe to see how a student keeps work and materials in order, especially when there may not be a clearly defined work space. The way that a student writes and colors on paper, worksheets, or workbooks gives you another indication about organization. Keep in mind that writing and coloring on paper in a two-dimensional space is strongly affected by visual-perceptual skills. Does the student always start on the left and work toward the right? Is there a discernible pattern to how subject matter is arranged on the paper when drawing and writing? Another important aspect of organization has to do with keeping routines and schedules. Every teacher has a set of rules for maintaining order in the classroom. Can the student remember these rules and respond to cues for quiet during assemblies, for instance, or remember that PE is before lunch but after study hall?

Examples of Problem Solving and Organization

Language arts finishes and Sharmane now must record her daily science experiment observations for growing three plants in different light conditions. This is the fifth day of measuring the growth of sunflower seeds, but Sharmane still forgets the necessary materials to complete the task. She has lost her ruler and borrows one from a friend. Then she measures each plant but has forgotten her notebook to record the observations. After retrieving her notebook, she forgets her first measurement and starts over again. She proceeds to record her measurements in the wrong daily column, negating all her efforts. As you watch Sharmane's behavior, you begin to wonder about perceptual problems, especially when you observe that she is holding the ruler upside down. You speculate that her disorganization may be the result of visual-perceptual problems and you wonder if color coding the plant containers and corresponding boxes in her notebook would be an immediate help to getting Sharmane through this assignment.

You are still observing Nathan in PE class. He blows up as soon as someone else picks up the ball that he has just kicked across the gym. It is obvious that his organization and problem-solving skills are at a very basic level. His poor impulse control detracts from any organized problem-solving approach, even at the level of what to do if someone takes what he wants. However, you note again that Nathan can figure out what to do with his body to kick accurately but that he does not follow verbal directions and is not able to tell you what he wants to do. For instance, he can get the ball out from under the chair without tipping the chair over and can throw the ball through a shortened basketball hoop. He really likes Station 2 and throws the ball through the hoop over and over again. You notice his organization for this activity and speculate about the effect of the right sensory information on his performance.

Posture/Motor and Visual/Motor Skills

The last two categories on the observation form, posture/motor and visual/motor more directly tap into areas of expertise for therapists. We encourage you to review our discussion about their educational relevance (see tables 2.2, 2.3, and 2.4 in chapter 2). The particular questions we have posed on the form can be readily answered by observing students in school activities. To describe a student's ability/disability profile in detail will require additional observation and assessment.

Observe the student's posture while at rest for seat work and while moving around the classroom and school. Of course, the most functional posture for using hands and eyes together skillfully to play or write is upright; however, many students with severe motor involvement cannot assume this posture without adapted equipment and, in fact, may need assistance even to change their position. The key is to observe how a student's posture facilitates engagement in the task at hand, whether it be looking at a toy, feeding oneself, playing a musical instrument, or using a computer keyboard. Watch for signs of adequate energy and stamina for the task. Slumping postures, wandering attention, shortness of breath, fatigue, and even falling asleep indicate that the student's schedule and activity roster may need to be revised.

Watching a student handle small objects, such as scissors, pencils, crayons, and rulers, will give you an immediate idea of grasp and release patterns and skill level. If you observe problems, you must further assess and observe the student to determine why the problems exist. Does low muscle tone contribute to wrist instability? Perhaps poor tactile discrimination provides inadequate feedback about the shape and texture of the object handled. Remember to share your observations with other team members in language that makes sense to them. In addition to looking at grasp, release, and manipulation when students draw or write, look at the final product. Very light lines or heavily drawn lines indicate problems with muscle tone and joint stability or motor planning of the hand and forearm. Overall legibility results from visual-perceptual abilities, including well-spaced and well-formed letters and words. Reviewing a student's written work and drawings can provide important clues, even when you have not seen how the work was produced.

Examples of Posture/Motor and Visual/Motor Skills

You observed that Sharmane slumped across her desk when doing her language arts exercise. Now you watch her carefully as she records her science experiment observations and note that she has an immature grasp, does not use adequate wrist extension, and writes only 20 words in two minutes. You wonder about her coordination and ask her teacher what Sharmane does in recess. You learn that Sharmane never uses the playground equipment and dislikes PE class. Most of the time she sits and talks with another girl and watches everyone else run around. One final observation provides other clues for your analysis of her performance in the classroom. Sharmane takes her weekly spelling test and then copies next week's words. You look at the two lists and are amazed at the difference in legibility; that is, the form and spacing of the letters. Her legibility was much improved on the list of words she copied, rather than those written from memory. This makes you wonder about her visual-perceptual skills, in addition to possible problems with muscle tone and motor planning. Now that you have watched Sharmane "in action," you have a good idea of where you need to begin with your assessment.

You have just watched Nathan race around the gym with no sign of fatigue. Mr. G. says that this is what Nathan is like all of the time. After watching Nathan shoot baskets and drop-kick the football, you don't have concerns right now about muscle tone and motor skills. In fact, you know Nathan has excellent gross motor skills for a five-year-old. You watched carefully, too, as he consistently dribbled the ball and shot baskets with his right hand, indicating that he prefers his right hand as the lead and uses the left to assist when needed. You decide that you want to see how Nathan behaves in the classroom to get a better idea of his attention span and sensory processing skills in more structured tasks, so you schedule another time to see him.

Conclusion

The first component in our model of school-based therapy is analyzing the student's performance during school lessons and activities. This is accomplished by translating how students' abilities and deficits affect how they participate in the classroom and other areas of the school environment. We have followed two students, Sharmane and Nathan, as they participated in school activities and we have observed some strengths as well as problems that they have with completing their tasks successfully. Our observations have led to speculation about what may be contributing to their problems during academic lessons and physical education.

You may feel that you know just what to suggest for Nathan and Sharmane based on what you have learned about them thus far. However, if you do begin intervention now, your opportunity to provide effective consultation is dramatically reduced. Before making any intervention plans, especially ones for other team members to carry out, you should consider the other two components of our consulting model: the knowledge and experience of a student's family, teachers, and other specialists; and how the school environment promotes or reduces performance. Once you have gathered this information, you will be ready to sit down with your team members to generate desired educational outcomes and interventions appropriate to the specific roles and responsibilities of the other team members.

Selected Readings

Baumgart, D., L. Brown, I. Pumpian, J. Nisber, A. Ford, M. Sweet, R. Messina, and J. Schroeder. 1982. Principle of partial participation and individualized adaptations in educational programs for severely handicapped students. *Journal of the Association for the Severely Handicapped* 7(2):17-27.

This article describes the principles of ecological assessment and illustrates how to view a child's performance on a task within the context of the environment. Depending on the environment in which the task is performed (home, child care, or school), performance expectations for the same child may vary.

Cook, D. 1991. Functional behavior assessment for children with sensory integrative dysfunction. In *Pediatric service delivery,* edited by W. Dunn, 35-74. Thorofare, NJ: Slack.

This resource is an excellent observation guide for physical and occupational therapists to rate the impact of sensory integrative deficits on self-care, behavior, approach to new activities, touch, memory, school activities, academic work, gross motor, perceptual fine motor, and sensory motor integration.

Dunn, W. 1991. Forms for analyzing sensory and motor characteristics of task performance. In *Educating children with multiple disabilities,* 2d ed., edited by F. Orelove and D. Sobsey, 67-75. Baltimore: Paul H. Brookes.

This simple form provides a guide for viewing motor performance during any task. It focuses on muscle tone, physical capacity, postural control, and movement characteristics.

MacDonald, C., and J. York. 1989. Assessment of student participation in general education class. In *Collaborative teams for students with severe disabilities,* edited by B. Rainforth, J. York, and C. MacDonald, 256-57. Baltimore: Paul H. Brookes.

This observation guide focuses on assisting students with severe disabilities to participate in classroom routines and activities and highlights social and communication skills.

In addition, the following forms for assessing performance in school are excellent and are available in Lessons 1 and 9 of: Royeen, C., Ed. 1992. *Classroom applications for school-based practice.* Bethesda, MD: American Occupational Therapy Association.

Motor checklist for occupational and physical therapy (Mary Barler)
Functional mobility/self-help assessment (Arlene Wesley)
Classroom materials checklist (Merriam Struck)
Feeding sample worksheet (Gloria Frolek Clark)

Figure 3.1

Observing Student Performance in School

Student: Sharmane Age: 8 years Date: October 1

Observed by: Martin Shaker, OT

Activity observed: Filling out reading worksheet and recording science observations

The following questions provide a framework for observing a student in school. The focus of the questions is on behavior and skills that are viewed by educators as essential for successful performance in school.

Performance Parameters	Comments
A. Purpose of Task 1. Academic or nonacademic subject or area? 2. Objective of lesson/activity? 3. Relationship to student's IEP goals/objectives?	Subject: Language arts and science Objective: Complete reading worksheet. Record data about experiment. IEP currently being developed
B. Nature of Activity 1. Individual, paired, or group? 2. Therapeutic domains (motor, perceptual, neuromuscular, sensory processing, adaptive behavior)? 3. Sensory input inherent in task?	Individual activities focusing on fine motor and perceptual domains, visual input for reading and spacing science data in columns, touch/proprioception for holding and manipulating pencil and ruler.
C. Accuracy of Performance 1. Which parts of task can student do? 2. Which parts are difficult? 3. Does student compensate? How?	Answered 3 of 7 questions on worksheet while others completed it. Lots of erasures and false starts. Watches other children for cues. Doesn't record data in correct columns; forgets notebook; loses ruler. Correctly identifies which plant grew the most.
D. Attention to Activity 1. Length of attention to task? 2. Distracted? By what stimuli or event? 3. Can refocus attention if interrupted?	Writes for only 1 minute before wringing hands and then looks around and starts talking. Follows lead of other children—if they start writing so does she. Is most distracted by talking and movement of classmates.
E. Handling Transitions 1. From one activity to another? 2. Within areas of the classroom/school? 3. Has previous activity affected performance?	Easily switched from reading worksheet to science experiment but is distracted equally during both. Moves around a lot more during second task (science). Looked around during first task rather than moving.

Performance Parameters	Comments
F. Problem Solving 1. Understands and follows directions? 2. Has plan of what to do? 3. Makes changes if difficulty arises?	Doesn't ask teacher for help but relies on peers—borrows ruler, looks at what others are doing. Appears to know what end result is expected but can't complete task smoothly.
G. Organization 1. Desk, cubby, backpack (3-D space)? 2. Papers and workbooks (2-D space)? 3. Knows schedule and class routines?	Desk is stuffed with books, folders, and crumpled paper. Couldn't find ruler. Asked 3X what comes after science.
H. Posture/Motor 1. Comfortable, upright posture for seat work? 2. Functional self-help and playground skills? 3. Adequate energy and fatigue levels? 4. Gets around school environment adequately?	Slumps over desk. Teacher reports Sharmane avoids playground equipment and dislikes PE. Likes to sit and talk with friends.
I. Visual/Motor 1. Uses age-appropriate grasp (pencils/crayons)? 2. Uses objects (scissors, erasers) with skill? 3. Draws/writes legibly with even force and spacing? 4. Uses dominant/assist hands appropriately?	Immature pencil grasp—no wrist extension or open web. Too much pressure on pencil. Uses right hand consistently with left as assist. Legibility much improved when copying letters. Writes 20 words/2 minutes.

Impressions:
(Summarize observations, identify any further assessment needed, outline recommendations.)

1. Has problems with sequencing parts of task herself but watches other students for cues. Models their behavior accurately.
2. Assess visual-motor integration and motor planning skills.
3. Check out muscle tone and pencil grasp. Try slant board for writing tasks.

Figure 3.2

Observing Student Performance in School

Student: Nathan Age: 5 years Date: March 15

Observed by: Natalie Morris, PT

Activity observed: Adaptive PE gross motor centers

The following questions provide a framework for observing a student in school. The focus of the questions is on behavior and skills that are viewed by educators as essential for successful performance in school.

Performance Parameters	Comments
A. Purpose of Task 1. Academic or nonacademic subject or area? 2. Objective of lesson/activity? 3. Relationship to student's IEP goals/objectives?	Subject: Adaptive PE Objective: Develop ball-handling skills as identified on IEP
B. Nature of Activity 1. Individual, paired, or group? 2. Therapeutic domains (motor, perceptual, neuro-muscular, sensory processing, adaptive behavior)? 3. Sensory input inherent in task?	Paired task within group activity focusing on gross motor and perceptual domains. Heavy pounding/movement in running, kicking, etc. Distracting auditory input.
C. Accuracy of Performance 1. Which parts of task can student do? 2. Which parts are difficult? 3. Does student compensate? How?	Good kicking and coordination; avoids being hit with ball; knows how hard to throw to hit target; efficiency and control decrease as Nathan appears to become overstimulated.
D. Attention to Activity 1. Length of attention to task? 2. Distracted? By what stimuli or event? 3. Can refocus attention if interrupted?	Activity increases dramatically as period progresses; can't attend to directions or modeling; keeps going over to pile of mats to jump.
E. Handling Transitions 1. From one activity to another? 2. Within areas of the classroom/school? 3. Has previous activity affected performance?	Runs from one center to another, especially if ball rolls away. During walk to PE he was touching everyone and everything.

Performance Parameters	Comments
F. Problem Solving 1. Understands and follows directions? 2. Has plan of what to do? 3. Makes changes if difficulty arises?	Oblivious to verbal directions. Gets mad if someone takes "his" ball. Can figure out how to get ball from under equipment without tipping it over.
G. Organization 1. Desk, cubby, backpack (3-D space)? 2. Papers and workbooks (2-D space)? 3. Knows schedule and class routines?	Nathan moves easily thru the gym but needs much greater structure to stay on task in a large area.
H. Posture/Motor 1. Comfortable, upright posture for seat work? 2. Functional self-help and playground skills? 3. Adequate energy and fatigue levels? 4. Gets around school environment adequately?	No signs of fatigue; good ball skills; does not pace himself. Really needs to calm down before returning to classroom.
I. Visual/Motor 1. Uses age-appropriate grasp (pencils/crayons)? 2. Uses objects (scissors, erasers) with skill? 3. Draws/writes legibly with even force and spacing? 4. Uses dominant/assist hands appropriately?	Dribbles ball and shoots consistently with right hand. Uses left hand as assist. Need to see him perform fine motor activities.

Impressions:
(Summarize observations, identify any further assessment needed, outline recommendations.)

1. Enjoys motor activity but is easily overstimulated by movement and noise. Seeks pounding and heavy touch/pressure. Needs external structure to define activity.
2. Explore with teachers ways to alternate fast-paced gross motor activities with calming ones in defined space; that is, under mat or play tug-of-war while sitting.
3. Give Nathan something to carry (ball bag) on the way to PE to focus him during walk through halls.

Chapter 4 focuses on the second component of our model of school-based consulting—the human resources involved. Specific topics discussed include how to:

- identify professionals and family members as critical members of the consultative experience
- learn about professional members' expertise and prior experiences with consultants
- identify family members' expertise and experiences as well as their concerns and goals
- understand professionals and family members' expectations about the consulting interaction

At the conclusion of each section, some sample questions or conversation starters are suggested as guides to refine your consulting skills.

Chapter 4

Identifying Human Resources

We need a shared view of what is going on . . . our hopes for the future, what is going well for us, what not, what we want to do about it, and so forth—a moving mosaic of information . . . We have to free ourselves up to explore, discover, learn, create, and plan together . . . This seems more likely if we make all data valid, acknowledge our differences, and agree to put our energy into working the common ground.

Weisbourd 1992

Consulting therapists work more effectively with school specialists and family members when they understand the backgrounds, expertise, and experiences of each team member. While your goal is to become as well informed as possible, you must carefully elicit needed information in an unobtrusive and friendly manner. If these are new relationships, team members may be anxious and you definitely do not want them to feel as if they are being "grilled." On the other hand, most team members will feel respected by your interest in their backgrounds and experiences. Understanding team members' perspectives is the cornerstone for the joint development of an effective plan to meet a student's special needs.

What are some of the topics about which you might want information in order to work effectively with this team? You want to know who are, or should be, members of the team. What is the knowledge base and prior experience of the professional team members? What experiences have family team members had with other consultants and systems? What concerns and goals do both family members and professionals have for the student? What are the teacher's classroom rules, routines, and preferences? What are the family's preferences for your conduct in the home and at school? Finally, what kind of follow-up does each member expect? We will discuss each of these issues separately.

Identifying Key Personnel

Most of your students will have both general education and special education teachers. Depending on the needs of the student, the team may have some or many other specialists, such as occupational therapists, physical therapists, nurses, physical education specialists, instructional aides or assistants, psychologists, and speech-language pathologists. In some situations, other special teachers may be instrumental in a student's education; for example, art, music, or shop instructors. Sometimes the specialists may not even be in the school but are members of the community; for instance, the YMCA recreation program leader, a religious official, or a nonschool-based professional, such as the student's pediatrician. Coordinating a comprehensive implementation plan requires you to make sure that all major professional and family members are included. Coordinated implementation is impossible if all the key players have not been identified. Not only does coordination facilitate planning and program implementation, but it saves the family time and effort. Many times parents are asked to explain their concerns in separate conversations with teachers and therapists over and over again. What is the appropriate role for the student?

Questions about Identifying the Intervention Team

1. Who are the teachers and instructional assistants who work with this student?
2. Who are the parents, siblings, grandparents, and other caregivers who should be members of this team?
3. Are there other specialists who are involved with this student?
4. Are there any others (including the student) who should be members of this team?

Professionals' Knowledge Base

There are some professional team members about whom you will need more information than others. The people you should focus on are those professionals who will implement your suggestions, such as the general and special education teachers and other therapists. Try to get a sense of their disciplinary training. In what philosophy or frame of reference were they trained; for example, Piagetian, Montessori, neurodevelopmental, or sensory integration? What kind of certification do they have (for example, registered occupational or physical therapist, licensed clinical social worker, learning disabilities teacher, or general educator)?

Often professionals will have special expertise that can benefit a student or family. For instance, knowing that a teacher is familiar with a specific learning style or that a physical therapist has expertise with prosthetic design will help you develop your consultation plan. The most important information is what experience each team member has had with children who have disabilities similar to those of the student for whom you are providing services.

In addition, some team members may have valuable expertise outside of their professional domains. Perhaps a new student teacher has a younger brother with cerebral palsy and brings a wealth of personal expertise to the team that is unrelated to her professional training. Sometimes knowing about a team member's hobbies or other avocations can help you match students' needs and professional team members' interests. If you recommend fine motor activities for a preschool student and know the child's teacher enjoys sculpting, you might suggest an activity involving clay or papier-mâché. Likewise, knowing that a second grade teacher has a black belt in karate provides a basis for discussion about movement, learning, and self-esteem.

Understanding team members' disciplinary knowledge as well as their work experience will help you make informed choices about your interaction as a consulting therapist (see chapters 6 and 7 for further discussion). Team members may have graduate training in their discipline but little experience working with students with certain diagnoses. The reverse might also be true—they may have a wealth of experience but lack formal knowledge about etiology, symptoms, and intervention strategies. For example, an educator with a Ph.D. in educational psychology had little experience teaching children with pervasive developmental delay but was knowledgeable about current theories and research. However, her classroom assistant led a Boy Scout troop that included a child with this diagnosis. Although the assistant could handle the student's behavior, she did not understand the neurological basis for his learning problems. Obviously, this educator and assistant have different roles, experiences, and knowledge; the consulting therapist must consider their individual needs for information and follow-up to assist the student with achieving the desired outcomes.

Questions about Professionals' Knowledge

1. I've learned that special education teachers sometimes have different perspectives about teaching and use different approaches. For example, some teachers use a more structured approach, such as behavior management, whereas others rely on open education approaches. What is your preference? Are there other aspects about your training that would be helpful for me to know about?

2. I heard that you conducted a workshop for the district's special education professionals on cued speech last year. I've always been fascinated by cued speech and am looking forward to learning from you while we work together. What other specialties do you have that are related to teaching?

3. I know that you've been teaching for—what? Twelve years? You've developed quite a lot of expertise in those years. What techniques have you found that usually work with students who have needs and strengths similar to Nathan's?

4. You were holding Liu in such a supportive position during lunch that it looked like second nature to you. Obviously you've had experience with positioning techniques before Liu joined your class. Can you tell me about your experiences with students with physical disabilities?

Professionals' Experiences with Consultants

A strong influence on the success of your consultation is the team members' prior experiences with consultants in general and with consulting therapists in particular. A team member might have worked with a consultant whom she considered to be a long-lost sibling because they communicated so well. On the other hand, a team member might have had terrible experiences with consulting therapists and concluded that they always act as if they know more than the other team members. Some may have been bossy or others simply not helpful. Each of these scenarios affects how team members will feel about you as you begin the consultation process. You should discern early on how each team member views consultation. You can be a very successful consultant no matter what the prior history but understanding a team member's reaction to prior experiences with therapists is definitely an advantage. If a team member has had close relationships with other consulting therapists, you can build on those successful experiences. If prior experiences with consulting therapists were negative, you can identify why and learn from those mistakes.

In order to develop a positive relationship, you should also find out what the team member thinks of consulting as a therapeutic tool and what the person believes is the underlying philosophy of consulting. One parent might be very enthusiastic and another may be skeptical that consulting can have positive results. One teacher will be relieved if you pull out the student for therapy, whereas others will prefer therapy activities integrated into the classroom curriculum. The point here is not that you always have to accommodate each teacher's preferences; obviously, your decisions about how to provide intervention will be based on what will facilitate reaching student outcomes. However, knowing as much about the expectations and desires of each team member can facilitate your communication and help you establish common ground.

Interviewing team members can be a little tricky. You want to learn about their backgrounds and expectations without appearing to be interrogating them. Interviewing skills are discussed in chapter 6, which focuses on the stages of consultation and the interpersonal skills needed in each stage. Remember that most people like to talk about themselves if their conversation partner is honestly interested and receptive.

Questions about Professionals' Prior Consulting Experiences

1. Have you ever worked with a physical or occupational therapist?
   a. If yes: Tell me how it went.
   b. If no: Let me tell you a little bit about physical therapy as I see its role in education.
2. Have you worked with therapists as consultants? How did that go? What were the best things about the experience? What would you like to have changed?
3. What were the benefits of having the occupational therapist work with Chuck right in the classroom? Were there any drawbacks?
4. What do you think would make our consultation really work for you?

Family Members' Experiences

Families are integral members of the student's team. They will be involved in planning for the student's special education and related services, monitoring the program, and evaluating the outcomes. Some family members may carry out some of the education or related services. You should consider family members as team members just as you consider other colleagues as team members (Lillie and Place 1982).

Families enter into the consulting relationship with prior experiences with professionals and service systems. These experiences will influence their thoughts and feelings about you and will be particularly influential during the initial stages of your relationship. The choices that you make about interacting with family members should be based on your knowledge of their experiences, beliefs, and attitudes.

Knowing about a family's experiences with their child's special needs is important information. Is this an only child and the parents have no prior experience with children at all? Maybe the student is in tenth grade and the parents know a great deal about their child's special needs. You might approach these two families very differently based on their prior experiences and knowledge.

Understanding a family's prior experiences with service systems is also important. Families who have been involved in finding specialized medical and child-care services will probably have had good and bad experiences. Specific knowledge about what happened will be useful for you as the consulting therapist. Follow up global judgments or statements, such as, "Well, Brady's PT has been very helpful but we've never seen an OT before." You need to know specifics. How does this family define *helpful*? People often describe services as being helpful when something specific happened that made things better for the student and/or the family. What was better for this student and family as a result of interacting with the physical therapist? What did the physical therapist do that the family interpreted as helpful? Do they have any ideas about what an occupational therapist might contribute? If the PT provided direct service in the outpatient department of the local hospital and you now recommend consultation in the classroom, expect to spend time discussing how your approach will achieve desired outcomes.

Parents may or may not have had experience with the consultation model. They may fear that consulting means the student will receive less or inappropriate services. Other families may have previous experience with consulting therapists and you will want to determine if these experiences were positive or negative and why. Inquiring about these experiences and attitudes can assist you with communicating more effectively.

As you explore issues about consultation, be prepared to review with the family the reasons why consultation was chosen as an appropriate service delivery technique. Perhaps you know of other families who expressed concerns initially but have been impressed with the results of consulting. You might want to ask those families if you could refer another family to them to talk about consultation. After you initially identify a family's experiences, make plans to continue to receive feedback from them about their experiences.

Questions about Family Members' Experiences with Therapy

1. I know you're a librarian, Ms. Dunkins. I want to understand what you already know about Tourrette's Syndrome so I can explain the role of occupational therapy in treating this syndrome.

2. A physical therapist saw Joaquin in the baby clinic for three years. Would you give me some ideas about what physical therapy activities he enjoyed and how they helped him? What else would you like me to know about your son?

3. Have you ever worked with a physical therapist? Let me tell you about what we do in school to help children learn.

4. How did Charlie's therapist work with him last year?

Team Members' Concerns and Goals

Each student's program should reflect the concerns and goals of the family as well as the professionals. If parents are to assume their rightful role as active partners in decision making, professionals must make the effort to inquire about and include the family's recommendations in the plan. Open discussions about desired outcomes can foster parent satisfaction and will facilitate evaluation of the effectiveness of the educational program.

You must also clarify the concerns and goals of all the key professionals working with the student, including your own. As the consulting therapist, you may have your own prioritized goals for a student; however, if they are not congruent with those of the primary service providers, the goals are not likely to be met. As discussed in chapter 1, the nature of consultation is to work through others. You may go into a classroom and be concerned that the student is not using the proper pencil grip. This concern may be of minor importance to the teacher right now who is more concerned that the student is very messy at lunch, which results in a lot of teasing. Due to the student's inefficient eating skills, she takes a long time to eat so she frequently misses playground time. If you come in to the classroom with a writing program, the chances are that this teacher will not be very receptive to your suggestions. If you take the time to find out what the teacher's primary concerns and outcomes are and then bring up yours, you might well be able to incorporate some of the fine motor exercises you want in a self-feeding program. That way you can address your goals while satisfying the teacher's concerns. There may be times when this merger of goals is not as feasible. In those cases, you need to make some thoughtful decisions about which goal is more critical for the student at this time. Clear identification of the outcomes and concerns of professionals is the first step in effective intervention plans.

Questions about Team Members' Concerns and Goals

1. Mr. and Mrs. Mikulski, as you know, we are talking about what we want Sheila to be able to achieve by the end of this school year. We've spent a lot of time talking about positioning and exercises. I know you have given a lot of thought

to what you want her to do. You told me at our last meeting that you would like her to take off her own coat. Can you tell us some other things you would like her to learn?

2. I'm very interested in what you want for Nathan. Can you tell me what's important to know about working with him and you? What do you hope he'll learn to do next?

3. Thanks for inviting me into your classroom to observe William, Mrs. Padrillo. What concerns you about William? You have said that he seems to be very clumsy. What does he do that seems out of the ordinary?

Classroom Etiquette

Webster's dictionary (1971) defines etiquette as, "(1) The forms, manners, and ceremonies established by convention as acceptable or required in society, in a profession, or in official life. (2) the rules for such forms, manners, and ceremonies" (p. 337). We chose this term to describe how a teacher expects (knowingly or unknowingly) others to behave in the classroom. Experienced teachers usually have some very well-defined expectations, yet even new teachers have some expectations. Some points of etiquette are common sense; for instance, do not talk about a student when the student or others can overhear. Some rules may be idiosyncratic to the teacher or other professionals. The best ways to find out the teacher's "rules" are to ask and observe. Remember, even after you have asked about how to conduct yourself in the classroom, there may be an unspoken etiquette that you can detect only by careful observation. For example, a teacher may say that he does not mind if you sit on the students' equipment while observing children at the playground. But careful attention shows you that after observing playground activities the teacher seems very tense and does not look you in the eyes when you try to share your observations. This is odd because usually this teacher is very open and receptive. You might be more observant about the teacher's behavior on the playground to see if there is some unspoken rule you may be unknowingly violating. We have developed some common etiquette guidelines that may be helpful to you.

When you first arrive in the classroom, it is essential that you do not violate class rules. Much of what is appropriate is common sense, but some expectations are unique to individual teachers. Ask the teacher how you should act while observing students and while providing therapy in the classroom. Listen carefully to what is said and what is implied and then respect the preferences of the teacher and professionals. Table 4.1 (page 56) lists suggestions to make your initial observations less intrusive. Strategies for interacting in the classroom on a regular basis are recommended in table 4.2 (page 56).

Table 4.1
Classroom Etiquette: Suggestions for Initial Observations

1. Never talk about the student when the student or others might overhear your discussions.
2. Conduct yourself as a welcomed and privileged, but unobtrusive, guest.
3. Do your best to observe the student at a time when the target behavior is most likely to occur and at a time that is convenient for the teacher. Be punctual.
4. Ask the teacher if it is all right to take notes. Do not feel shy about asking because most teachers are receptive and understand the need to jot down observations.
5. Be as quiet and unobtrusive as possible. Stay out of the main action of the activity that you are observing, unless invited by the teacher to join the group.
6. As an observer, avoid engaging students in conversation. If students talk to you, respond briefly and direct them back to their task
7. Unless your presence would interfere, move to areas in which you can clearly observe what the student is doing.
8. Avoid congregating with other adults. Do not chat with the teacher or other professionals. Write down any questions you have and save them for later discussion.
9. Treat the equipment, the furnishings, and the environment with respect. Do not move furniture or change routines without first discussing your intentions with the teacher.
10. Always look for something positive to comment on when you share observations with team members.

Table 4.2
Suggestions for Ongoing Participation in the Classroom

1. Never talk about a student when the student or others might overhear the conversation.
2. Wear clothing appropriate to the activity and environment.
3. Note the posted schedules and follow class rules.
4. Ask for advice when working with any materials or equipment with which you are unfamiliar, such as computers, homework, or science experiments.
5. Encourage students to do their own work. Avoid giving answers to assignments or making models for students to copy in any medium unless this is a part of your intervention plan.
6. Sit down with the students so that you are at their level when communicating.
7. Talk quietly, as appropriate, and target your sentence structure and length to the developmental level of the student.
8. Implement interventions during naturally occurring school routines and activities.
9. Help children be successful during cleanup and transition times.
10. Be alert to what is going on in other parts of the classroom so that you will know when help is needed.
11. Avoid unnecessary conversation with other adults in the classroom and on the playground.
12. When you have doubts about a procedure or the student asks for permission to do something unexpected, say to the student, "Let's ask the teacher."

Questions about Classroom Etiquette

1. I'd like to take some notes while Angel is in the gym. Would it bother you or the other students if I discreetly jotted them down?
2. I saw Michael hit Lisa with a block yesterday. How would you prefer that I handle the situation when I see students misbehaving? Should I intervene or would you like me to come get you or Ms. Hill?
3. Lea seems to have taken a shine to me. Every time I join the language circle to observe, she comes to sit in my lap. This doesn't interfere with my observation, but I wondered what you thought of it. Does this distract the group? Should I discourage her?

Family's Etiquette

Just as teachers have expectations for people in their classrooms, families have expectations about the behavior of others in their homes or about their interactions with others. Each family has its own culture and defines what it considers appropriate. You show respect for a family by finding out the family's rules of etiquette and abiding by their expectations.

One of the crucial pieces of information you need to find out first is the family members' modes of communication. Are some members of the family non-English speaking? If so, is there a trusted family member who can translate or do you need to bring an interpreter with you? Are there special adaptations that you need to make in order to communicate effectively? A grandparent who has difficulty hearing might understand better if you face the individual or sit closer when talking. Are there cultural factors that influence communication? Some families may avoid direct eye contact when talking with professionals (McCormack 1987; Lynch and Hanson 1992).

Some family members may feel that you are being overly familiar if you address the parents by their first names, whereas others might think you are distancing yourself if you never use their first names. Some families have expectations about who should talk when and to whom. Decision-making strategies also vary among families. Appreciating each family for its unique culture and strengths will make you a valued member of the partnership you have established to meet the student's needs.

Another critical consideration is to identify family expectations about planning and providing services and try to accommodate these preferences. Family-centered practices have been developed for early intervention and should serve as models for schools as well (Hanft et al. 1992, Sparling 1992). Some families might want only the parents to be involved in the student's special education whereas others may want to involve relatives and friends. The best way to find out who the family would like to assist them with planning and assessing their child's education is to ask them. Every effort should be made to accommodate their desires. If this is not possible, you will at least understand the family's preferences for services and will have begun a partnership between the school and family.

Questions about Family's Etiquette

1. Ms. Rozza, I know that you want Emil to drink from a cup. I can come out to your house on a Thursday, my day for home visits, or you can come to school to meet with me. Which would you prefer?

2. I noticed at the last IEP meeting that you translated the test results and other information for Joey's grandfather. Translating for him while talking with all of us is really hard! We have a teacher at school who speaks Spanish fluently and frequently translates for families. Would you like her to translate for your father so you won't have to do both jobs at the same time?

3. You mentioned that you were beginning literacy classes at the high school. That's great! I know you're very interested in Imi's walking and I wanted to share her program with you. What's the best way to do this? I wish I had more time, but I can call you only about every two weeks. Would it be helpful if I jotted down short notes? Can you tell me the words that you can already read? If you would like, I can give you a list of words to take to class and work on so that you can read my notes.

Your Own Training and Experience

You should remember that you are a critical element of the team as well and that your experiences and knowledge will have an impact on the course of the consultation. As a consulting therapist, you will augment and add to the expertise of the other team members. What is your previous experience with consulting, with meeting the needs of students with specific learning needs, and with working in an educational system? Analyzing your own background will prepare you to be an equal partner in this relationship. Previous experiences, such as working in home health, may help you in your role as a consulting therapist. Acknowledging your strengths and professional development goals is an ongoing process. The appendix includes a questionnaire for you to use to continuously monitor your skills as a consulting therapist. This type of self-evaluation can be very rewarding as you develop or refine your consultation skills.

Conclusion

As a consulting therapist, you will be relying on other personnel to implement the intervention plan. Therefore, your understanding of the knowledge and experience of each team member will help you to individualize your interactions and expectations for each person. This attention to detail will enhance the possibility of success for any suggestions you make. As a consulting therapist, you will typically enter other people's settings to observe, participate, and evaluate. These settings might include a PE teacher's gym, a parent's living room, or a teacher's classroom. Remember to show respect for each team member by finding out and abiding by the person's etiquette rules and expectations. We encourage you to step outside yourself and try to adopt the perspective of the people with whom you will be consulting. To assist you in this endeavor, we recommend the materials in the selected readings section that follows.

Selected Readings

For insights into the teacher's perspective:

Ashton-Warner, S. 1971. *Teacher.* New York: Bantam.

This classic text gives you insight into the perspective of teaching based on joy and love. The story describes the philosophy of one teacher and recounts life in a Maori school in New Zealand. Reading the book is not only instructive but inspiring.

Bruckeroff, C. 1991. *Between classes.* New York: Columbia University.

An ethnographer studies the education setting and describes what teaching is all about by becoming a teacher for a year in a suburban high school.

Giangreco, M., R. Dennis, C. Cloninger, S. Edelman, and R. Schattman. 1993. I've counted Jon: Transformation experiences of teachers educating students with disabilities. *Exceptional Children* 59(4):359-71.

Sixteen teachers are followed throughout a school year as they include a student with severe disabilities full time in their general classrooms. Important points are made about consultation from therapists and other specialists. The title comes from one teacher's dramatic realization halfway through the school year that she is responsible for including the student with disabilities in class activities and cannot rely on the student's aide to do this for her.

Spindler, G. 1987. *Education and the cultural process.* Prospect Heights, IL: Waveland.

Stories from students, parents, teachers, and administrators are presented in this anthology of articles that describes the many variables and perspectives that influence school life.

For insights into the family's perspective:

Goodman, J., and S. Hoban. *Day by day: Raising a child with autism/PDD.* New York: Guildford.

A day in the life of two families who are raising preschool children with autism is depicted in this excellent video. The parents express their hopes and concerns as they go through their daily routines of caring for their daughters.

Lynch, E., and M. Hanson. 1992. *Developing cross-cultural competence: A guide for working with young children and their families.* Baltimore: Paul H. Brookes.

This book is an excellent guide for working with families from various cultures who have young children with disabilities. Highlights include a discussion of major cultural and ethnic groups living in the United States and recommendations to enhance the sensitivity of service providers.

McConkey, R. 1985. *Working with parents: A practical guide for teachers and therapists.* Cambridge, MA: Brookline.

This useful manual provides practical advice about why and how to work with parents individually and in groups. Quotes from parents are included to support or illustrate the author's recommendations. One chapter discusses how to develop working relationships with four types of families who may sometimes be more challenging to professionals than more traditional families. Other helpful chapters guide the professional in leading parent groups or courses and how to communicate effectively in written reports.

Simons, R. 1987. *After the tears: Parents talk about raising a child with disabilities.* San Diego: Harcourt Brace.

Several families share their experiences in intimate and powerful words in this book. Although this book was written to share parents' thoughts and feelings with other parents of children with disabilities, the stories can help professionals gain insight into the anguish and joys of parenting a child with disabilities. Therapists will benefit from the chapters in which parents share their perspectives about professionals and working with the school system.

Turnbull, A., and H. R. Turnbull. 1986. *Families, professionals, and exceptionality: A special partnership.* Columbus, OH: Merrill.

This comprehensive text provides information about the diverse complexities of families and individuals with disabilities throughout their life cycles. The book is a systematic and scholarly analysis of families; however, in the authors' words, "We have seasoned this book with a compelling real-life flavor. We undergird its theories and concepts with the reality of the living laboratory" (p. v). The book is written for an interdisciplinary audience. The chapters dealing with communication strategies, referral and evaluation, and parent participation in the IEP are extremely useful.

For insight about the student's experience:

Davis, R. 1994. *The gift of dyslexia: Why some of the smartest people can't read and how they learn.* Burlingame, CA: Ability Workshop Press.

Viewing dyslexia as a "gift," the author describes how his unique learning style allows him to visualize and see things from many perspectives. Although humiliated as a child learning to read and write, Davis is now an architect and educator.

Grandin, T., and M. Scariano. 1986. *Emergence: Labeled autistic.* Novato, CA: Arena Press.

In an autobiographical account of life with autism, Grandin offers fascinating insights into the daily experiences and family issues surrounding autism and discusses how her extreme sensitivity to sound and touch profoundly influenced her behavior.

Chapter 5 focuses on the third component of our model of school-based consultation, the environment, and provides you with information and practice to develop skills for analyzing:

- the supports and demands of the environment in which a particular student is expected to learn and perform
- the characteristics of the general school environment
- the sensory environment
- the specific learning environment

Chapter 5

Assessing the School Environment

The classroom. What memories does it evoke? Colors? Smells? Noise? Routines? Reading groups? YOUR DESK! The child who sat behind you, in front of you, beside you? Desks in rows? THE TEACHER'S DESK! The coat closet, the blackboard, the windows, the pencil sharpener, the bulletin board, the alphabet across the front of the room way up high above the blackboard . . .

Chandler 1992

In order to develop an effective intervention plan, you should observe the student while learning and performing in specific school environments. We recommend the following principles, which will be discussed in detail later in the chapter.

1. Observe the actual environment in which the student's target behavior is expected; for example, observe the child during lunch if you have been asked to assist with a feeding program or observe gym class if the target is improved coordination.

2. Observe the environment while the student interacts in the environment.

3. Keep your observations value neutral, systematic, and structured.

The following section focuses on analyzing the physical environment of the school and provides a framework for observing a student engaged in a school-based activity. You should determine which elements of the environment support or facilitate learning and which interfere with or impede learning. Ideally, you should analyze all elements of the student's school environment, including classrooms, gymnasium, cafeteria, playground, hallways and other transit paths, and bathrooms (if appropriate). If such extensive observation is not possible, coordinate with the teacher to observe the environment and activity that will provide the most useful information for a particular student. We recommend a strategy that begins with getting a sense of the general environment, then identifying the sensory environment, and finally analyzing the specific environment in which the student functions.

General environment—the overall structure, furniture, and equipment of the space in which the student performs. Observe the room arrangement, traffic patterns (how a student moves from one place in the room to another), and the routines that affect performance.

Sensory environment—auditory, visual, tactile/kinesthetic, and movement inputs. Observe the effect of lighting, proximity to other people, sounds, and types of textures on student performance.

Particular environment—the actual space in which a given target behavior is expected to be performed. This analysis addresses the boundaries of the space, the characteristics of the space, the necessary materials, the organization of the space, the demands of the task, and the opportunities for independence.

Principles

1. ***Observe the actual environment in which the student's target behavior is expected.***

   Understanding the environment is a critical factor in determining which elements influence a student's performance in school. The consulting therapist will benefit from observing the context in which the student is expected to learn and produce. A student's performance changes as the demands and supports of the environment differ. You can get the most information by watching a student as he or she actually performs in a particular school environment. For example, the teacher has requested assistance with feeding Celestine solid food. You will be able to obtain the most information about how the environment supports or detracts from Celestine's eating if you observe her in the environment in which she usually eats. Similarly, you will learn a great deal about Shep's attention behaviors if you observe him while he is in a place where attention is at a premium, such as in a small-group math session, rather than observing him in free play.

2. ***Observe the environment while the student interacts in it.***

   Just as environments influence students, students influence environments. Observing the student performing in a particular environment ensures that you have an accurate perception of it. Let's say that you have been asked to assist a teacher with a student's impulsive behavior. You have never met this teacher before, so you stop by her classroom before school to get a sense of how it is organized. You walk into a room that is quite organized. All of the crayons are sorted into orange juice cans by color, the dramatic play equipment is stored in labeled and distinct spaces, and the unit blocks are arranged in geometrically precise arrangements. Depending on your expectations, you might think, "Oh, brother, do we have a problem here!" However, if you came in 45 minutes later when the students were present, you might draw very different interpretations about the demands and supports of this environment. You would see students setting up a grocery store and serving customers. You would see play food on the shelves of the climber, students lying on the floor pencilling signs for the store, and a student building a cash register with building blocks that he had dumped on the carpet next to the climber. Your conclusions would probably be very different if you see the students performing in the actual environment rather than just the classroom without students.

3. ***Your observations should be value neutral.***

   Your own personality will affect your impression of the classroom in the above scenario. If you like very organized and structured places, you might be happy with the scene before the students arrive and horrified by the goings-on after they arrive and influence the environment. On the other hand, if you like unstructured activities, you might be pleased to find the students having so much freedom of choice and activity in this classroom. In either case, you have drawn an incorrect conclusion. How can both perceptions be wrong? The most important goal is to observe the student's actual performance and how the environment enhances or inhibits that performance. Environments by themselves are value neutral. What might entice you or drive you crazy is of minimal importance compared to how a particular student is influenced by an environment. You can serve the student best by consciously stepping outside your own preferences and determining the pluses and minuses for the student to whom you are responsible.

4. ***Your observations should be systematic and structured.***

   A reproducible form, School Observation: Environment, is included in the appendix for recording your observations. This form is intended to supplement your discipline-specific evaluations by providing a systematic way to observe the school environment from a neutral perspective. The form is divided into three sections, which are discussed in detail below. The first section focuses on the general environment and provides an overview of the learning infrastructure in which the student performs. The second section looks at the specific sensory environment and focuses on the stimuli that affect the student's performance. The process concludes with observation of a specific space in the school environment in which the student's performance can be observed. This last observation entails a microanalysis of the demands and supports of the environment.

Figure 5.1 (pages 64-66) shows a completed form for observing the environment. Please refer to this figure as you read the text that follows, which discusses each section of the form in detail. You will find a blank School Observation: Environment form on pages 145-147 of the appendix that you may reproduce and use. To complete the practice exercises in this chapter, you will need to make a copy of this form. Then select one particular student and environment to observe as you work on the practice exercises.

Figure 5.1

School Observation: Environment

Student observed: Nathan Age: 5 years Date: February 18

Activity: Adaptive PE Environment observed: Gymnasium

The following questions help identify environmental factors that facilitate or interfere with learning. Observe all relevant spaces of the student's environment, such as classrooms, gym, cafeteria, bathrooms, playground, and hallways.

Observation of the General Environment

Room Arrangement	Observations
1. Room size and shape adequate for task?	(Yes) No — 4 stations (perceptual-motor) Large, unobstructed gym
2. Furniture/equipment arrangement?	Diagram room on back of sheet
3. Varied space available?	Intimate 6″–18″ Personal 1½′ – 4′ (Social 4′–12′)
4. Space for personal belongings?	Describe: N/A
5. Active and quiet spots?	(Yes) No — Space is available for quiet time but it's not clearly marked off

Traffic Patterns	
1. Clearly defined pathways?	Yes (No) — Nathan has to be led from one station to another
2. All areas and materials accessible?	Yes (No) — Water fountain blocked by equipment
3. Any architectural barriers?	Yes (No)
4. Time and distance student covers.	Describe: 3-minute walk from classroom to gym

Routines	
1. Adequate structured/unstructured time?	Yes (No) — Large space promotes distraction and wandering
2. Toileting, drinks, snack?	(As needed) Scheduled

Observation of the Sensory Environment

Auditory	Observations
1. Sounds in and out of observed setting?	Describe: Lots of echoes, kids shouting
2. Unique acoustical features?	Carpet (Cinder block) Other: no windows, high ceilings, wood floor

Visual	
1. Adequate light?	(Yes) No Source: ____ Natural ✓ Fixtures
2. How is color used?	Highlight Guide Background Other: Walls and floor similar color—no variation
3. Intense glare on materials?	Yes (No)
4. Unique visual features?	Describe: Stations look very similar.

Tactile/Kinesthetic	
1. Flooring	Tile ____ % Carpet ____ % Other 100 % wood
2. Use of textures in furniture/materials?	Describe: Pretty "hard" environment
3. Light touch from others?	Describe: Large space limits bumping into one another
4. Unique tactile features?	Describe: Mats piled up are a big attraction for jumping.

Movement	
1. What movement/breaks are permitted?	Describe: Almost too much movement! Need defined breaks.
2. Who moves through this space and how efficiently?	Describe: PE class of 8 children; random movement despite centers.
3. Unique movement features?	Describe:

Observation of a Particular Learning Environment

Intent of Space	Observations
1. What is this space intended to facilitate? Gym allows large movements; 4 motor centers could use more structure.	Learning, resting, playing? Fine motor, **gross motor**, language, academic, social, self-help? Perception Independent, **cooperative**? Pairs Intent unclear?
2. Clear boundaries?	Yes **No** Need pathways defined.
3. Enough space?	**Yes** No
4. Necessary materials easily accessible?	**Yes** No
5. Materials/furniture enhance performance?	Yes **No** Centers are numbered but children do not respond.
6. Time student is seated and/or in same position?	Time: N/A Seated ______ Same position

Recommendations for improving student performance:

1. Set up a quiet area marked off by carpet squares to rotate through after each center to keep Nathan from getting overstimulated.
2. Put feet or tape on floor to show path from one center to another.
3. Mark centers with different color flags or banners to help define them.
4. Incorporate mat area, since it's such an attraction, but provide structure; for example, crawl under mat on way to one of the stations.

Observation Guidelines

Before you begin to analyze the environment, collect information about the student and the environment that will facilitate your observation, recordkeeping, and report writing. Included on the School Observation: Environment form are spaces for the student's name, date of observation, the activity to be observed, and the environment to be observed. Noting the time of day is also helpful since some students show a pattern of optimal behavior depending on the time of day; for example, if a student comes to school hungry, her behavior might be better after she eats a snack or lunch. You may want to note the activity that preceded the observation and where it occurred; for instance, a given student might perform better after a rest period or a quiet activity while another student may excel after gym.

Observation of the General Environment

When you first enter the environment, take a moment to get a general impression of the environment. How is this space set up? What is the shape of the room, including placement of permanent fixtures, such as the lights, windows, and doors? How is the furniture arranged? Take a few minutes and sketch the room plan on the back of your observation sheet to help you when you later analyze all of your data and develop recommendations. As you look around to get a general sense of the environment, keep in mind that your goal is to determine how these elements affect the student's performance. However, don't hesitate to step back to try to take the perspective of the student and decide, "How do I feel about this room? Why would I be comfortable here? What might cause me problems?"

Once you have a general sense of the room, identify the traffic patterns used by the students as they move through the space. Sometimes defined paths may look reasonable, but then you see students constantly taking a shortcut that disrupts another area. How much time and effort is expended by the students as they move through these environments? Are there hazards or distractors that might create impediments, such as architectural barriers? What are the cues, such as color coding, signs, or colored tape pathways, that assist with movement in this particular space?

Students respond well to spaces that are suited to the expected behaviors. Some activities may be supported by engaging in small groups whereas others are best performed alone. How does the environment support varied activities? Students of all ages respond better if they have a chance to vary their activity level—just look at the sensory-laden behaviors exhibited by participants at a day-long workshop. The ideal situation is to vary concentration with physical activity. What opportunities are facilitated by changes of pace in this environment? Are these opportunities available as your student needs them or are they on a prescribed schedule? If so, how does this schedule seem to meet the needs of your student?

Students feel supported and safe if they have a place for their own things that is defined and protected. One way that adults in schools show their respect for students' individuality is by providing a space for their personal belongings. How does the environment you are observing deal with this fundamental need? Are there cubbies or lockers? Do the students keep their school supplies and personal belongings in their desks? What about lunch boxes and bulky coats and boots?

Once you have a good sense of how well the overall environment is working, identify how school routines and schedules assist or impinge on your student's performance. Examine as many routines as possible. How are toileting breaks handled? What are the procedures for snack and lunch? Does your student have to move between or among different classrooms? How structured is the daily classroom routine? Remember that structure is value neutral. You might judge the environment as chaotic but may observe that this student not only copes with the variety but actually thrives on it. Conversely, a very structured routine may be precisely the level of structure that allows another student to succeed. Routines and structures may assist or interfere with a student's ability to stay on task, to attend and perform, and even to show up for an assigned task on time.

Practice Exercise

Choose a classroom that you would like to learn more about. Copy the observation form in the appendix and complete the first section to assist you with systematically collecting data about the environment.

Observation of the Sensory Environment

The sensory environment provides supports or distractions for learning. Understanding these inputs is essential to analyzing how and why students react in the ways that they do. Auditory, visual, tactile, and movement stimuli are all important. Some suggested guidelines for observation are included in this book, but you may identify others that are equally as important in your situation.

Auditory Input

How loud is the general noise level and does it appear to distract the student? What is the source and intensity of the background noise? How well does sound carry in the room?

Visual Input

Which visual cues does your student rely upon to assist with performing specific tasks? Some classrooms use color or texture to provide cues and others use pictographs or words; for example, a sign that reads, "Reading Corner: Quiet Voices" or a picture of students reading by themselves provides useful cues. Are there significant visual distractions? Is there glare or unwanted light that might affect the completion of paperwork? One of the mistakes that is often made in this analysis is to evaluate visual impact based on the observer's position. The light may glare on the blackboard at the student's eye level but be quite comfortable from the adult's position. Make sure you do your best to see what the student experiences.

Tactile Input

How does the tactile input affect a student's attention? Are there a variety of textures available for sensory input? What are they and how does the student appear to benefit or be distracted by them? Is the student vulnerable to jostling from other students? What is the student's reaction to expected and unexpected touch?

Movement Input

It is important to determine what movement occurs in the room, who is moving, and how efficiently the movement occurs. First analyze the necessary movements of the student you are observing and then analyze the effects of other students' movements in this space. What movement is permitted in the space? What movements actually occur, whether permitted or not? How does the movement affect the student's performance? Keep in mind that some students move because it helps them stay on task. Sample observations follow.

Celestine's teacher has asked you for assistance with keeping Celestine on task while she completes her math work. You observe that she is seated with her back to the traffic path to the pencil sharpener. Just as she becomes interested in the math assignment, someone walks behind her, bumping her seat and distracting her. In this situation, other students' movements interfere with Celestine's performance. Consider another situation, where movement is facilitative. Stephen becomes restless and fidgety when he has to sit for an extended period of time. Once he loses his place, he begins to interfere with the other students and soon attracts the negative attention of the teacher. The consulting therapist observed that when Stephen was given the opportunity to move just a little (to throw away a paper, sharpen a pencil, or get a drink of water) he could stay on task much longer.

Practice Exercise

Move on to section 2 of the School Observation: Environment form and analyze the sensory impact of the environment you are studying.

Observation of a Particular Learning Environment

The final aspect of the environment to consider is the specific space and time in which the student is expected to learn and perform. The observation form will help you collect information about the supports and demands of the particular situation. Some of the elements that you might want to consider include the boundaries, characteristics, and organization of the space; the needed materials; the demands of the task; and the opportunities for independence.

Clear boundaries may be of great importance to some students and unnecessary for others. Boundaries indicate acceptable behavior for a particular space; for instance, library areas are clearly not suited for messy art projects. If students are expected to keep the puzzles in the manipulative area, are there clear boundaries marking where the manipulative space begins and ends?

Some rooms are hampered by the fact that they do not have enough room for the activity to be performed. Students with physical disabilities may be unable to enter some spaces because of crowded conditions. Some students who distract easily may be overwhelmed by too many materials too close at hand.

On the other hand, some spaces, such as lunch rooms or gyms, might be cavernous and negatively affect a student. Part of your environmental analysis includes determining the effects of these huge spaces on the student. How does a student follow instructions during PE class? Does the student have difficulty hearing instructions outdoors on a windy day or because of echoes inside the gym? If such is the case, the space may be creating additional difficulties for the student and result in poor performance.

Is the space clearly organized? Are the materials available to accomplish the desired task? If not, how is the student's performance affected? Some tasks require the use of a pencil and a worksheet. Once an assignment is given, does the student have to go to her desk and get a pencil then go to the teacher's desk to retrieve her workbook? If so, does this offer an impediment (by limiting the time the student has to work on the actual task) or a distraction (by requiring too many consecutive tasks) to the student? For some students, this type of movement will actually serve as a performance enhancer because the movement then allows the student to settle in for some concentrated thinking.

How much time is the student required to participate in a particular activity and what are the impacts of this requirement? Students who need frequent position changes might experience fatigue if an activity is too long. However, a string of very brief activities might not give a certain student the necessary time to concentrate and sustain attention. Your decision about the appropriateness of the length of the task would be better supported if you could see the student before the targeted behavior observation. If this is not possible, a detailed conversation with the teacher or the assistant might provide needed insights.

If the teacher tells you that Juan has a particularly hard time staying alert and attending during the final reading exercise, you will learn the most about how to assist if you can observe him during that time. Ideally you would want to observe what occurs prior to that time also. Perhaps Juan was moved from his supported wheelchair to a corner seat so that he could sit with his peers during the lesson. You might observe that since this exercise is at the end of the school day, Juan is fatigued. While he could tolerate sitting in the corner chair earlier, he is just too tired to do so later in the day. The physical demands make him irritable, which he expresses by acting out. If you had observed Juan early in the day, you may well have missed this easily solved problem.

Finally, our society values independence. How does this particular environment foster or inhibit the student's independence? Are all the equipment and supplies needed by the student accessible (for example, pencil sharpener, drinking fountain, toilets)? Are there contributions you can make to enable the student to be more independent?

Practice Exercise

After you have completed the final observation about the specific environment, review all the data you have collected about the environment you are analyzing. Try to identify how the environment influences the performance of a particular student. Once you have determined these patterns, what recommendations might you offer to enhance the environment? Some suggested readings are offered at the conclusion of this chapter if you need further information upon which to base your recommendations. Once you have analyzed the environment, write your recommendations in jargon-free language to convey this information to the teacher. Be prepared to share the rationale for each of your recommendations based on your observations and data collection.

Conclusion

Knowing the general environment, the sensory environment, and the characteristics of the particular environment in which the student is expected to perform, you are now in a position to analyze the demands and the supports available to the student. You can summarize this information and share your insights with the teacher and other team members. You might report, for instance, the environmental factors that make it possible for Celestine to succeed and those that distract her. This analysis will be an invaluable source of information to plan for Celestine's success. After discussions with the team members, you can then suggest how to maximize this student's performance in the particular or general environments.

Selected Readings

Chandler, B. 1992. *How to design and implement classroom programming.* In *Classroom applications for school-based practice,* edited by C. Royeen, Lesson 3. Rockville, MD: American Occupational Therapy Association.

Practical guidelines are provided for therapists who consult in schools. Several sections focus on the inanimate and animate environments. Numerous examples demonstrate how to effectively modify school environments.

Dunn, R. 1988. Research on instructional environments: Implications for student achievement and attitudes. *Professional School Psychology* 29(1):43-52.

Dunn, R. 1992. Redesigning the conventional classroom to respond to learning style differences. In *Hands-on approaches to learning style: A practical guide to successful schooling,* 42-47. New Wilmington, PA: Association for the Advancement of International Education.

These two articles focus on how the school environment (including lighting, room arrangement, carpeting, and temperature) affects students' learning and behavior, whether or not they have a disability. Teachers are strongly encouraged to use movement, tactile, and kinesthetic input within their instruction to enhance learning and are cautioned against letting students sit too long for uninterrupted periods.

Jensen, E. 1994. *The learning brain.* San Diego: Turning Point Publishing.

This informative book summarizes more than 200 current neurobiological and psychoeducational studies. Written in user-friendly language, the author speculates on the implications for learning for each study and suggests "Best Bet Resources" for additional readings. One of the 16 chapters focuses on how aspects of the general environment (clothing, lighting, seating and posture, aromas, heat, noise, visual input) affect brain function and learning.

Merrill, S., Ed. 1990. *Environment: Implications for occupational therapy practice.* Bethesda, MD: American Occupational Therapy Association.

This innovative collection of articles examines the role of the environment in facilitating performance from the perspective of sensory integration theory. Individual chapters are devoted to itinerant school therapy as well as pool therapy, psychiatry, and the neonatal intensive care nursery.

Roley, S. 1991. Sensory integrative principles and playground design. *Sensory Integration Special Interest Section Newsletter* 14(1):1-6.

This article discusses considerations for designing an imaginative and challenging playground. It covers the target population, using natural landscape, the design team, safety elements, and meeting children's play needs through equipment and structures.

Somer, R. 1969. *Personal space: The behavioral basis of design.* Englewood Cliffs, NJ: Prentice Hall.

This interesting text describes the interaction between the environment and human behavior. The chapter Designed for Learning uses research to identify the connection between the classroom setup and students' behaviors. Therapists may also be interested in the scholarly review of hospital spaces included in the chapter Designed for Refuge and Behavioral Change.

Chapter 6 focuses on:

- decision making in the role of consulting therapist
- intervention strategies needed to achieve the student's educational outcomes
- consulting methods for translating your knowledge to assist other team members
- interaction styles selected to establish and maintain optimal relationships with team members

Chapter 6

The Therapist's Role in the Consulting Process

> *Social roles are learned as men and women acquire the culture of their group, although roles may become so much a part of the individual personality that they are played without awareness of their social character. Roles are not people; they are the parts played on the social stage, and they can be analyzed separately just as the drama can be considered apart from the performance and the performers.*
>
> Rose 1970

You review the student's records, observe the student in the classroom, and give specific recommendations to the teacher immediately. Is this good consultation? That depends. We believe that consultation usually works best if the actions are jointly agreed upon. However, there may be mitigating circumstances which suggest that you choose a different strategy. What if you observe a student in a physically threatening circumstance? Would you give the teacher explicit instructions about how to hold the student so that the student is no longer in danger? Given this situation, you would choose to act directly and emphatically.

However, let's look at another scenario. What if the teacher was reading a book to a small group of students and you notice that Chuck is having difficulty staying on task? Do you interrupt the group and say, "Mrs. Martinez, please move Chuck next to you since he can pay attention better if he leans against the wall while looking at the pictures you are holding"? Or do you make a note to discuss this recommendation with Mrs. Martinez later? Assume you choose the latter. At the meeting you note that while Chuck is still having a hard time attending, the changes that Mrs. Martinez made have started to show progress. You support the intervention methods she is using by reminding her, "Chuck is sitting on the carpet square now instead of wandering around the room." You encourage her to continue implementing the program the team has designed to support Chuck's participation in the group and you remind her of Chuck's need for specific visual and tactile cues.

The purpose of this section is to describe the decisions that consulting therapists might make as they assist teams with identifying student needs and developing and implementing intervention programs. There are many aspects by which you define yourself. How you define your role as a consulting therapist will influence the way you interact with team members to address a particular student's needs. The most important part of this role definition is to consciously make decisions about how you will interact with team members. While much has been written about consultants' roles (see the selected readings list at the end of this chapter), our purpose is to help focus your decisions, strategies, and interaction style as a consulting therapist in the school system.

IEP Planning Decisions

Educational teams must make a number of decisions to determine how best to achieve student outcomes. Figure 6.1 illustrates the IEP planning and consultation role decisions that must be made before intervention begins. While the educational team decides which related services will enable a student to benefit from special education, therapists have responsibility for clinical decision making and must choose their frame of reference to guide assessment and intervention for a school setting. Therapists must answer the questions related to student outcomes and services (questions 1-4) with the education team and carefully consider team members' responsibilities and learning styles in order to decide how to implement consultation when appropriate (questions 5-6). The six questions must be answered in order, beginning with identifying desired student outcomes and concluding by determining an interaction style to assist team members with implementing therapeutic recommendations.

Figure 6.1
Flow of IEP Planning and Consultation Role Decisions

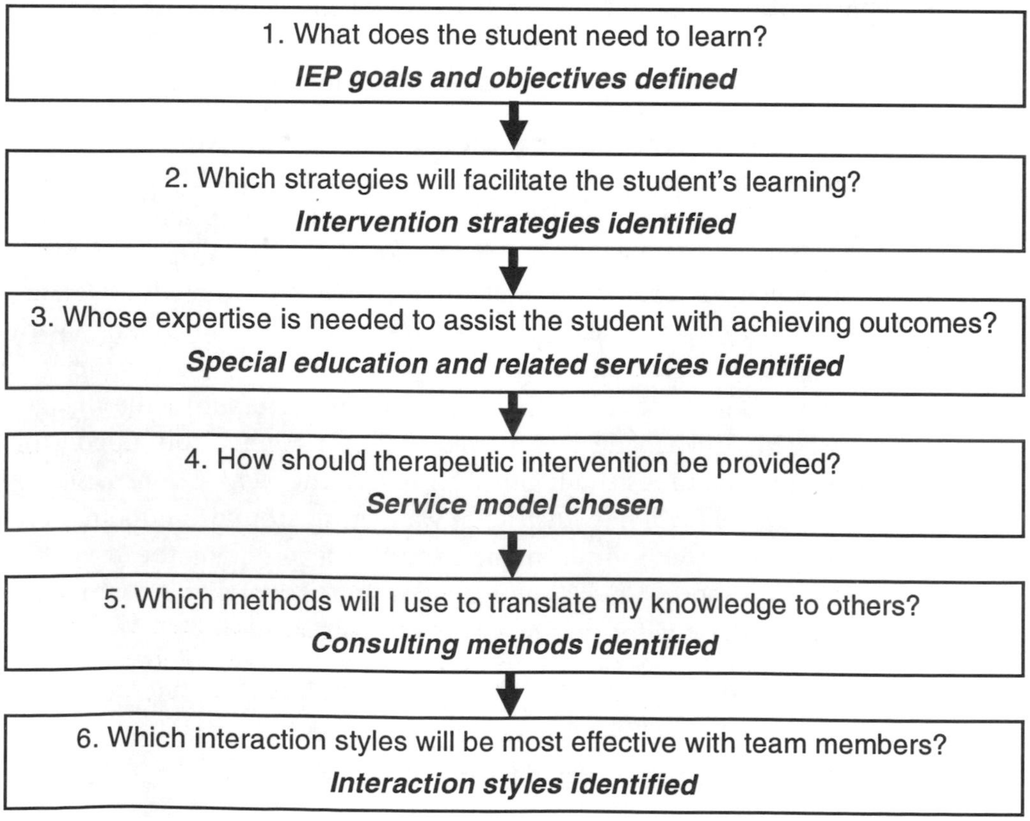
1. What does the student need to learn?
IEP goals and objectives defined
2. Which strategies will facilitate the student's learning?
Intervention strategies identified
3. Whose expertise is needed to assist the student with achieving outcomes?
Special education and related services identified
4. How should therapeutic intervention be provided?
Service model chosen
5. Which methods will I use to translate my knowledge to others?
Consulting methods identified
6. Which interaction styles will be most effective with team members?
Interaction styles identified

1. ***What does the student need to learn?***

   This is a crucial question since outcomes should guide all intervention. Posing this question to the team should lead to a discussion about educational outcomes and eventually result in identification of IEP goals and objectives. In order to talk knowledgeably about a student's learning needs and development, therapists may need to complete discipline-specific evaluations. Choosing a frame of reference to guide the selection of appropriate evaluation tools and methods, including observing students in the school environment, is the therapist's responsibility and provides an important avenue for contributing therapeutic expertise to team discussions.

2. ***Which strategies will facilitate the student's learning?***

   Outcomes describe desired behavior. Once the team knows the student's educational "destination," they can identify which strategies will help accomplish each outcome. We refer to intervention strategies as the options therapists employ when consulting with team members to achieve student outcomes. For example, if the outcome for a second-grade student with traumatic brain injury includes writing four sentences within five minutes during language arts, then what intervention strategies will help the student achieve this goal? Are a slant board and pencil grip needed to compensate for an immature pencil grip? Should the classroom environment be modified by providing the correct desk height and chair to facilitate eye-hand coordination? Can the teacher use a kinesthetic writing program to teach cursive?

3. ***Whose expertise is needed to help the student achieve goals and outcomes?***

   Therapists are often asked whether a student needs physical or occupational therapy before the team has considered which outcomes are desired (question 1) or which intervention strategies would be most effective (question 2). The response that almost always follows is "yes" or "probably" since therapists are very good at thinking of ways to enhance a student's development. However, the response could change dramatically if the question were rephrased as, "Is the expertise of an occupational or physical therapist necessary to assist a particular student with reaching a specific educational outcome?" For example, consider Tony, a seven-year-old boy with severe cerebral palsy resulting in delays in balance, fine and gross motor coordination, and oral-motor skills. Does Tony need occupational or physical therapy? Thinking of all the problems Tony has may lead you to automatically answer yes. How would you respond if asked whether physical or occupational therapy was needed to enable Tony to use a computer (the intervention strategy which will assist him to reach his educational outcome of communication with peers and participating in daily instructional activities)?

   Team members other than physical or occupational therapists may very well possess the expertise needed to assist Tony with using a computer. While the physical or occupational therapist contributed to the team discussion that led to the identification of the outcome, this expertise may not always be necessary to achieve the outcome. However, if the team decides the expertise of either or both therapists is needed, the therapists must choose a frame of reference to guide intervention recommendations and activities in the school setting, which is similar to the clinical decision-making process used to select evaluation methods. This leads to the fourth decision—how can the therapist's expertise be best employed to help the student reach the specified outcome?

4. ***How should therapy services be provided?***

   Once the educational outcomes, intervention strategies, and disciplinary expertise have been determined, the next decision should be how the service is to be provided. Which model would best help the student achieve desired outcomes? Most of the models identified in the professional literature (integrated therapy, consultative, and monitoring), include a consultation component as we have defined it.

   The exclusive use of either direct service or consultation is ineffective and violates the IDEA mandate for individualized services for students. While the use of a consultative model alone can help achieve certain student outcomes, direct intervention by the therapist, particularly in a separate space, should always be paired with some form of collaborative consultation with other team members. Students must function at home, in child-care settings, and in school; however, school clinics and therapy spaces provide only selected views of a student's performance. Therapists can avoid this narrow perspective by expanding direct service to include consultation with other adults to carry out their responsibilities and interactions with students in their natural environments.

5. ***Which method will I use to translate my knowledge to others?***

   Questions 5 and 6 relate to the use of a consultation model in which the therapist analyzes how to assist another adult with student-related responsibilities. The term *method* refers to the way in which therapists choose to translate their knowledge and expertise to others through instruction, modeling, demonstration, and support. The crucial determination is how best to help other people with their responsibilities and concerns, not teach them to be therapists. If a student needs a therapist to do the intervention, then direct service should be provided. When consulting, therapists must figure out how to use their knowledge and experience to assist other team members in their interactions with the student. This is one of the delicate considerations that makes consultation so different from and, in some ways, more complex than direct service. It is often easier to provide the therapy yourself than to figure out what the parent, teacher, or child-care provider needs to know and then pinpoint how to help them implement appropriate strategies to assist the student.

6. ***Which interaction style will be most effective with team members?***

   This final question relates to your skills in communication and interpersonal interactions. Depending on the situation and personalities of your team members, you may choose from a variety of approaches, ranging from expert to collaborative consultation. Therapists should adapt to various environments and the needs of staff and parents. If you can choose from a variety of interactional approaches, you will be able to adapt to different situations, as described below.

Identifying Your Consulting Role

The answers to questions 2 (strategies), 5 (methods), and 6 (styles) are the most relevant to your decisions about the role you will adopt for each consulting situation. Table 6.1 summarizes the essential aspects of your role: the intervention strategies you choose, the methods you select to translate your expertise, and your interaction style.

Table 6.1
Summary of Role Decisions: Strategies, Methods, and Styles

Decision	Examples of Choices
Which intervention strategies (actions to meet a student's needs) can best achieve desired outcomes for a student?	• assist the team member to acquire new skills • introduce a new resource or adapt existing materials • modify the environment • reframe the team member's perspective • change the routine or schedule of the student or the team member
Which methods (actions to translate consultant's knowledge to team members) will best achieve the desired outcomes?	• modeling • direct instruction • peer resources • encouragement • print or video resources
Which interaction style (how the consulting therapist communicates with team members) will best achieve desired outcomes?	• tell • sell • teach/advise • encourage or support

Based on these three elements, we propose the S/M/S model for consulting therapists: Strategy/Method/Style. Each of these elements is dealt with in more detail below.

STRATEGY → METHOD → STYLE

Strategies

Remember Nathan from chapter 3? After completing your assessment of Nathan, you decide that he would benefit from the application of sensory integration principles to help him concentrate in the unstructured environment of the gym. You believe that Nathan would stay on task longer if he were not overstimulated in the gym. You speculate that the intervention strategy to best accomplish this goal is to change Nathan's routine; for instance, do some relaxation activities with him that incorporate deep touch and pressure at the beginning of gym class. This change in routine represents the strategy (the first element of the S/M/S model) by which you hope to achieve a specific educational outcome for Nathan—improved performance in the gym.

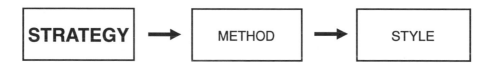

Some commonly used strategies are to assist team members with acquiring new skills, introduce a new resource or adapt existing materials, modify the environment, reframe the team's perspective, and change the routine or schedule. You will need to use a variety of strategies to meet the unique needs of your students. Consider Adam, a student with cerebral palsy whose desired educational outcome is to feed himself. You choose an adapted spoon and make him a splint to improve his grasp of the spoon (introduce a new resource). Finally, you teach the assistant the *Minnesota Feeding Program* (assist staff with acquiring a new skill). These are the strategies you will employ to improve Adam's performance and meet his educational outcome. Table 6.2 summarizes some common strategies and provides examples of each. Of course, you will develop other strategies to help your students achieve their educational outcomes.

Table 6.2
Intervention Strategies

Strategy	Examples
Assist the staff or family with acquiring a new skill.	• Show the teacher how to transfer a student without bending over. • Teach the parent how to position the child on the floor so they can play ball together. • Instruct the assistant in how to check a student's skin for rubbing and abrasions.
Introduce a new resource or adapt existing materials.	• Add nonskid material to the wheelchair tray. • Introduce built-up pencils. • Buy specially designed scissors for a student. • Order a corner chair.
Modify the environment.	• Establish tactile cues for a student with visual impairment to find the water fountain. • Assist the teacher with reorganizing classroom materials to make them more accessible. • Move the student's desk to a quiet area of the room.
Reframe the team's perspective.	• Help the teacher realize that a student's visual processing problems, not lack of interest, are causing reading problems. • Assist with identifying developmentally appropriate reinforcers for students on behavior management programs. • Analyze a task and simplify it for the teaching staff.
Change the routine or schedule.	• Advise the teacher to break up in-seat work; for instance, asking the student to take the attendance to the office. • Identify when a student is most receptive to learning and assist staff with introducing the most complicated learning materials at that time. • Encourage the teacher to allow the student to move independently in the classroom by crawling but have the student use a wheelchair elsewhere in the school. • Collaborate with the teacher to reschedule the student's activities to limit time in the prone stander to 30 minutes.

Keep in mind that any proposed strategy is only your best guess until you try it out. As you interact with other team members, you may decide that a different strategy would be more effective for a particular situation. For instance, you may have selected a strategy that proves to be incompatible with the classroom practices or that underestimates the skills of a team member. Your selection of a strategy will be affected by your knowledge of and your relationship with the other team members. Often you will need more information regarding the student's needs or the team members' backgrounds before you finalize your choice of a strategy. When you have acquired the needed information, you can alter your strategies as needed. Your goal is to make a conscious selection from a menu of strategies.

Practice Activity

Make a list of strategies that were helpful to you or that you know have worked well for others. Table 6.2 listed examples of strategies that we often use in our own consulting. Fill in the form below with strategies that you have used or would like to practice as you consult. For example, the strategy might be to assist the teacher with acquiring new skills. Under the Examples column, you might note that you used this strategy successfully when you taught the gym teacher how to use inner tubes to improve a student's upper body strength and coordination.

Practice Activity: Intervention Strategies

Strategy	Examples

Once you have thought of ways to apply these strategies, we suggest that you identify others. You might talk with a supervisor or a colleague about strategies they have used to enhance students' performances in school through consultation. Some of the selections in the reading list at the end of this chapter will provide you with ideas for additional strategies.

STRATEGY → **METHOD** → STYLE

Consulting Methods

All team members have unique experiences and knowledge. As a consulting therapist, your responsibility is to translate your knowledge for the other team members so that they can share your perspective and carry out your recommendations. After selecting an intervention strategy to help a student achieve a specific educational objective, your next choice is which method will work best to translate your knowledge to educational staff and family members. Remember that as a consulting therapist your services will be provided indirectly to students through their teachers, classroom assistants, family members, or other therapists. Which method will work best to motivate and develop expertise in the other team members so that the educational objectives can be accomplished for the student?

Some methods that consulting therapists frequently use to translate their knowledge to team members include modeling; direct instruction of a team member; encouraging team members' behaviors; and providing therapeutic equipment, reading materials, or audiovisual resources. Table 6.3 summarizes some of the methods that might be used to translate your knowledge to another team member.

Table 6.3
Consulting Methods

Method	Examples
Modeling	• Feed a student at lunch time. • Demonstrate how to put long-leg braces on and take them off.
Direct Instruction	• Show the assistant how to monitor range-of-motion exercises for a student with juvenile arthritis. • Discuss the use of a prone walker, including how to position the student, where to look for pressure points, how long to use it, and for which situations and times of the day you would use it.
Encouragement	• Agree that using new equipment takes time and offer to review procedures as soon as possible. • Congratulate a teacher on successful interaction with a student who dislikes being touched.
Providing resources	• Lend a parent a video about positioning a child with motor delays. • Share journal articles on a topic of particular interest to a team member.

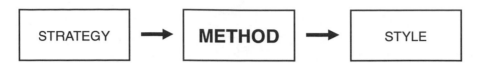

Modeling involves performing the behavior to be imitated so that the person you are trying to teach can see and observe it. Consulting therapists may demonstrate the desired activity and ask the staff or family member to imitate it. You may want to use modeling when your team member is uncomfortable or uncertain about how to begin the program or activity you have recommended. For example, you recommend that a student be positioned on a wedge but the teacher is hesitant to carry this out. Provide a model for the teacher by positioning the student yourself during circle time for several days. Once the teacher sees how quickly the student adjusts to this positioning device, the team member can then comfortably take over responsibility for your recommendation.

Direct instruction should be individualized for each team member. Some of the characteristics of effective training are:

- collaborative planning between you and other team members
- relevance of instruction
- uniqueness (meets the individual needs of the learner)
- flexibility
- clarity
- voluntary participation
- careful sequencing of learning tasks
- pacing the learner adequately
- selection of appropriate material to be learned
- recognition of the learner's comfort level

Gallesich 1982

Keep in mind that you do not always have to be the instructor. You might be aware that a teacher in another school supports a particular technique that you think will benefit Ronnie. You might arrange a meeting so that the experienced teacher can share his knowledge and enthusiasm with Ronnie's teacher. In another example, you might set aside extra time to give step-by-step instructions to a teacher as she learns a new skill and you help her to perfect the technique.

Encouragement is another method used by consulting therapists to translate their expertise for team members. Encouragement, whether planned or spontaneous, acknowledges that making changes in classroom routines and instructional strategies takes time and effort. You might convey your support by commenting, "It's only been three days since you began this feeding program and already Jake is drinking more juice!" In another example, while working in the classroom, you observe an aide interact effectively with a student and remark, "Joan, when you reminded Sylvia to use her slant board, her writing noticeably improved."

The final method that we often use to translate our knowledge to team members is to share information about available resources. As a member of another discipline, therapists have access to resources that may be unknown to educators and family members. You might inform a family member about resources on making a home accessible or tell a teacher about a positional device.

The methods you select will vary depending on many circumstances. Perhaps you know from past experience with a particular teacher that she likes to read about a new approach first and then try it out with your assistance. Perhaps another teacher prefers to talk about a new program with a peer who has had experience with it before trying it out. The methods you suggest should be individualized for each team member based on the specifics of commonly agreed-upon goals. Some of the elements that you might want to consider are:

- the context of the class, the school, and the school system
- the learning required to implement your recommendations (you might be introducing a new device to the classroom and need to teach the assistant to use it)
- the resources available to you (videos, reference material, manuals, time, other consultants)
- your own teaching style (for example, can you clearly break a task down verbally or are you better at giving a hands-on demonstration?)

Your own teaching preference should not solely determine the methods you choose to use with your team members. One of the best ways to identify which method to use to translate your knowledge is to ask the team members how they prefer to learn more about the intervention suggestions. Individuals may prefer learning methods that you can capitalize on. Some examples for inquiring about and suggesting methods follow.

Modeling: "I know you have some concerns about the students' reactions to Jimmy's new prosthesis. Would it help if I talked to your class for a few minutes about the prosthesis and answered the students' questions? I'm asking this question because I've always been someone who has learned from watching."

Direct instruction: "Mr. Stephans, look! The manual for Miguel's new keyboard just came in. Do you want me to look it over first and then explain to you how to operate it? OK. Can we get together for about 15 minutes before school tomorrow?"

Encouragement: "I admire your commitment to learn to use Adam's new computerized wheelchair. I'd be happy to show you how it works."

Providing resources: "I've discovered a great video about visual development that I found to be very helpful. I know you're interested in learning more about eye tracking. Would it be helpful if we viewed it together?"

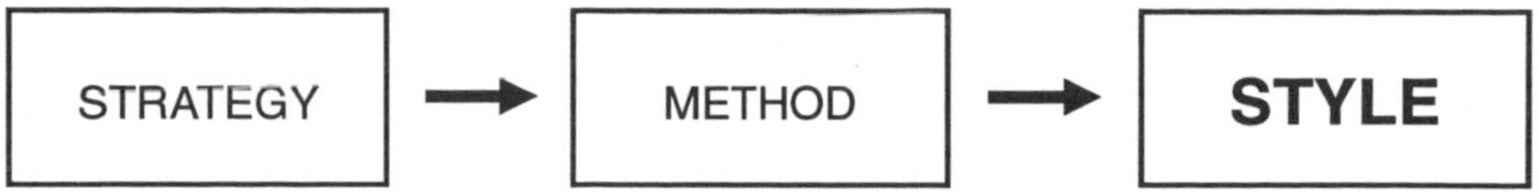

Interaction Style

Once you know the student's educational outcomes and have determined which strategies and methods to use, you must choose your interaction style—how direct you want to be when you interact with team members. Most of us tend to feel comfortable with a particular level of directness, which leads us to act in certain ways almost unconsciously. Perhaps you feel comfortable in an expert role in which you tell people how to best carry out your suggestions. Maybe you feel uncomfortable with this level of authority and would rather take a less visible role and use a supportive or nondirective approach in your consultation. When you consult, you must make overt choices about how to interact if you want to ensure a successful consulting relationship. Think about choosing your interaction style as planning a balanced meal. Dessert may be your favorite part of the meal, but you know you cannot rely on meeting all of your nutritional needs by eating pie. Likewise, you should have a continuum of interaction styles from directive to supportive so that you can select the style to match the needs of the consulting situation.

The two interaction styles presented in figure 6.2 depict two poles on a continuum of actions from most direct (telling people what to do) to least direct (offering an observation or reflecting on another's behavior). There are obvious differences between these two styles. When a consulting therapist tells a teacher exactly what to do and how to do it, she is assuming a very direct style of interaction. This style works well only when the consultant is viewed as an expert, has the authority to give directions, and knows that the instructions will be carried out as specified (Idol, Nevin, and Paolucci-Whitcomb 1994). On the other end of the continuum, if a consulting therapist praises and perhaps offers a new perspective, he is choosing to provide encouragement and support. This style usually occurs when all the parties agree to a given plan and the consulting therapist can encourage everyone to stick to the plan when complications arise or team members become discouraged. The importance of this interaction style should not be underrated because one of a consulting therapist's vital functions is to bring a new view or perspective to the situation and to keep team members motivated.

Figure 6.2
Opposite Poles of Interaction Styles

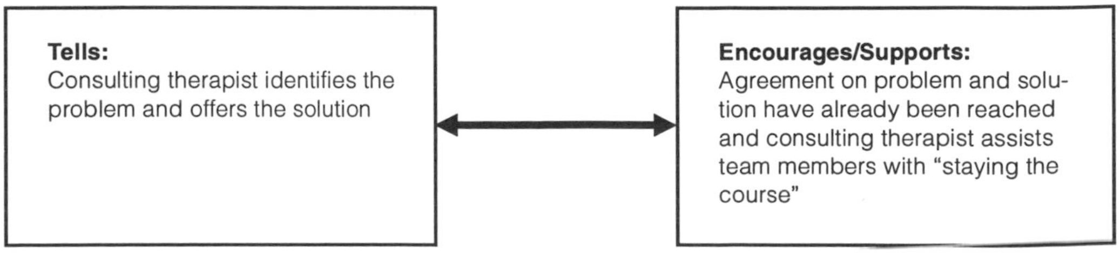

A wide range of interaction style options exists between these two extremes. Many researchers and practitioners have described and labeled points along this continuum (please see the selected readings list). For example, Lippitt and Lippitt (1978) identified eight roles:

- objective observer/reflector
- process counselor
- fact finder
- alternative identifier and linker
- joint problem solver
- trainer educator
- informational expert
- advocate

In a simpler model, Klein and Kontos (1993) identified three roles: prescriptive, co-active, and mediator. We have chosen four interaction styles to discuss: telling, selling, advising/teaching, and encouraging/supporting. We selected these four interaction styles because they seem to be the most prevalent styles that we have used in our consulting and because they represent discrete points on the interaction style continuum from most direct to least direct.

We have already mentioned the interaction styles of telling and supporting. A consulting therapist might also sell her perspective and recommendations when she is convinced that a certain instructional strategy would work for the student and the team member hesitates to accept the recommendations. Perhaps the team member hesitates because of lack of experience with the recommended technique or uncertainty about how to implement the program in the classroom. Conversely, a consulting therapist may choose to teach or advise when a team member fully understands the objectives but does not have the technical knowledge to accomplish the task. The therapist might teach the parent how to use a new piece of adaptive equipment or advise the assistant to avoid bending from the waist when transferring the student to a wheelchair. Figure 6.3 depicts the continuum of all four of the styles described in this text. The following scenarios demonstrate each of these interaction styles.

Figure 6.3
Continuum of Interaction Styles

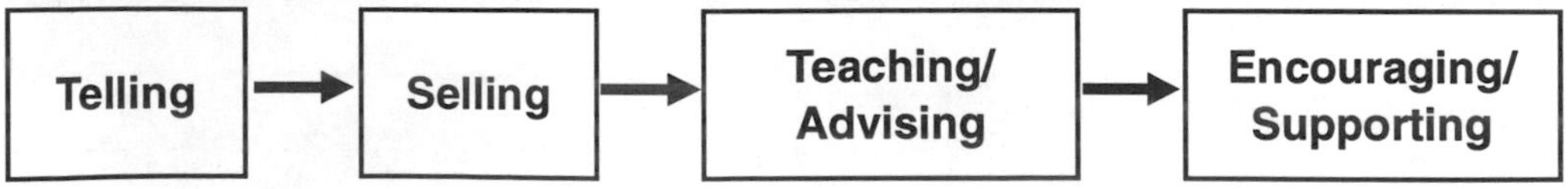

Telling

You observe Nathan on the playground in unstructured physical play when you see a fellow student kick a soccer ball wildly so that it flies over the fence and into the street. Remembering Nathan's overenthusiastic response to balls, you rush to shut the gate and intercept Nathan before he runs out to the busy street. You are concerned enough that you decide to be very direct with your recommendations. You approach his teacher and say, "I am concerned about Nathan's safety; someone left the gate open and he almost ran into the street. I believe we all need to be very vigilant with Nathan. I've observed that this is especially important when he's involved in physical activities. I wouldn't rely on verbal instructions or rules. When he gets excited he seems to forget all the rules and just runs on impulse. I'd like to look over his environments with you so we can identify potential hazards." You can tell that the teacher is relieved at your offer and eager to schedule an appointment to look at Nathan's environments with you.

Selling

You have been consulting with Mr. Zebrowski, whose student, Ray, has an attention span similar to Sharmane, a student with learning disabilities. Over the last few years, you and Sharmane's teacher have developed a system of visual cues about her schedule. You think this system will work well for Ray, also. When you offer this suggestion to Mr. Zebrowski, he is hesitant to try it for a variety of reasons. He thinks it might single Ray out, it might be too much work, and he's never had experience with anything like it, yet he is willing to learn more about the system. You set up a time when you and Mr. Zebrowski can observe Sharmane and then meet with Sharmane's teacher for 15 minutes in the teachers' lounge to discuss her positive experiences. Mr. Zebrowski is sold on the system and is willing to replicate it with Ray.

Teaching/Advising

Carole's mother tells you she is quite concerned about the way Carole sits when she is doing her homework. "She seems to lie all over the dining room table then just stops trying. Her teacher complains that she always has her head down on her desk and seems to tire very easily. Is there anything we can do to help her?" You have also observed Carole slouching at her desk with her feet dangling because they do not reach the floor. You advise her teacher to move Carole to a smaller desk and chair so that her feet can rest flat on the floor and you talk with her mother about putting a sturdy box under Carole's feet at home. You explain how these adaptations will provide appropriate back and leg support. A slant board will help keep Carole's wrist slightly extended with minimal fatigue and can be used at home and at school.

Supporting/Encouraging

Ronnie's team has agreed that he needs some calming techniques before beginning any academic task. His teacher wants to help Ronnie concentrate during the math lesson. You suggest that Ronnie listen to audiotapes with headphones while lying on a beanbag chair in a quiet corner of the room for five minutes before math. Meeting with the team two weeks later, the teacher expresses frustration. "He doesn't seem to be doing any better." You acknowledge that when you're in the "trenches" it is hard to see progress since it occurs slowly. You share your observations that Ronnie's time on task in math during your most recent observation is longer than the first time you were in the classroom. The teacher seems very pleased about this information. You suggest other ways to look for signs of improvement and methods for documenting these behaviors. She is pleased with these suggestions and with the signs of progress you have pointed out to her and she is motivated to continue with the intervention.

Practice Activity

During the next three days, try out an interaction style with a friend or family member. You may want to try to sell your husband on celebrating a winter holiday in Florida this year or encourage your 14-year-old daughter to clean up her room. If someone solicits your suggestions, try to tell them what you think they should do. You might teach a friend how to unclog a clogged drain. So take a chance, choose how directive you want to be for the given situation, and try one of the four interaction styles. Use the following form to record the reactions of the person you approached as well as your own impressions, including your level of comfort, how well the interaction style worked, and why it was successful or not.

Interaction Style Record Sheet

Interaction Style	Telling	Selling	Teaching/ advising	Encouraging/ supporting
Describe what you did:				
Describe the other person's reaction:				
Describe how you felt:				
Describe the outcome:				

Putting It All Together

As you have seen, selecting a role as a consulting therapist is very complicated. Your role is the sum of the elements discussed in the previous section—intervention strategies, consulting methods, and interaction styles. Your role may change from one moment to the next, depending on who is involved in the consultation and the context of the consultation. We will revisit our model of school-based consultation to guide you in selecting your role. The model suggests that you need to consider the student, the human resources, and the environment in order to select an appropriate role.

The Student

You start defining your role based on the student's needs and desired educational outcomes. Begin by asking yourself what each student needs to learn. If you can help students reach their educational outcomes with your therapeutic expertise, how will your services be provided; that is, what combination of direct therapy or consultation would be helpful? Each consulting situation requires you to learn about the environment and the human resources.

The Environment

The environment, as defined here, includes all school spaces, furnishings, and equipment that the students come into contact with, except for the human resources, such as teaching staff, family members, and peers. Analyzing environmental elements can provide excellent insight into how to proceed as the consulting therapist. Assess the environment to determine what physical supports might assist the student; for instance, equipment you might easily adapt, and what barriers prohibit the student from learning, such as inappropriate student seating. Analyzing the environment will help you to choose the best intervention strategies for improving the student's performance. The environment might also give you information about the preferences of teachers and other team members. The room arrangement, decorations, organization of supplies, and furnishings can provide hints about consulting methods and interaction styles to try. (Please review chapter 5 for a discussion of the environment.)

Human Resources

Most of the difficult decisions you will make as a consulting therapist will be affected by the complexities of human interactions. The greatest rewards of successful consultation can also come from interacting successfully with others to meet the student's needs. When selecting your strategies, methods, and styles, remember that you are almost certainly asking for behavioral changes from your team members who, in turn, will attempt to improve the student's performance. Try to figure out how you can least intrusively, but effectively, change attitudes and behaviors. You can gather ideas for consulting methods to try by observing how educators and family members interact with one another and with the student. Does the teacher use modeling or does she rely much more on verbal instructions? If you see her systematically reinforcing student behavior, you might use encouragement to help her learn a new skill. Does a team member seem interested in acquiring new knowledge or skills in general? Does she seek out a supervisor or a peer for advice? Is he the kind of person who can be found in the library looking up the latest research on a particular topic? Talk to team members about which methods they or other consultants have used that have worked well in the past.

You will also want to consider the personalities and styles of your team members as you decide which interaction style to use. Can you be direct and tell the person what you think needs to be done or should you step back a moment and offer encouragement? Remember to think about the suggested continuum of directness from telling to reinforcing/supporting. What information do you need in order to select your interaction style? The answers to all of the above questions depend on the desired outcomes for the student and the strategies you choose to use to accomplish these outcomes.

Let's say that you would like Akiba, a classroom teacher, to change the environment to accommodate a technologically sophisticated but bulky wheelchair. In our consulting model, this is the intervention strategy to improve student performance. You have noticed that Akiba relies on her fellow teachers as resources and you know a teacher in the school, Becky, who has successfully used a similar wheelchair with one of her students. Your consulting method will be to enlist Becky as a peer resource. Now, consider which interaction style you think would prove most successful with Akiba.

Perhaps you know Akiba well and recognize that you can ask her to call Becky to talk about the pros and cons of using this wheelchair. Maybe you decide you have to sell her on the idea of looking into this issue further so you leave her some literature and talk about Becky's satisfaction with using the wheelchair. Perhaps Akiba just does not understand why the chair would be helpful, so you decide to teach her more about posture and its impact on fatigue and performance. You think this information will motivate her to call Becky to find out more about it. Finally, you might need to acknowledge Akiba's concerns, perhaps about disrupting her classroom layout. During your conversation, you determine that she is also anxious about not being able to operate the wheelchair and worries that it might break down on a field trip. Once her concerns are acknowledged and she finds that you are supportive of her efforts, she may be able to call Becky to find out how Becky dealt with these concerns.

You can see from this example how your interaction style affects the success of a consulting plan. If you tell a teacher who has all of these unexpressed concerns to call another teacher about using the wheelchair, that call probably will not be made. On the other hand, a teacher who has used special equipment might not need or want this level of support for her feelings and concerns. When unsure of how direct to be, you are less likely to offend a team member if you choose to be less directive rather than more directive until you know the person's preferences.

Practice Activities

The best way to refine your skills is to practice them over and over again.

1. As a first step, you must be able to identify and analyze behavior change skills. Tomorrow, carry a small notebook in your pocket and practice observing people's behaviors. As unobtrusively as possible, jot down the methods or interaction styles that people use to change someone else's behaviors. Examples of these behaviors abound, not just in a consulting relationship.

   To simplify this task, try analyzing interaction styles first. Observe a situation in which one person wants another to do something. Is the person trying to sell, tell, teach/advise, or reinforce/support? How well did the approach work and why? Speculate how you would act in this same circumstance to produce the desired outcomes. Once you are comfortable identifying interaction styles, you can begin to concentrate on identifying the methods that people use; for instance, modeling, direct instruction, encouragement, and providing resources.

2. Now that you feel comfortable identifying the methods and interaction styles that people use, you can systematically practice them. At first, you might want to analyze a situation with a friend or family member. The person you choose should be your peer to simulate your work relationships with team members. Tell the person that you have been working on developing new consulting methods and interaction styles and ask for assistance with practicing these skills. Create a situation in which you both have to come to some conclusion; for instance, selecting a movie to see that night. Try out a variety of consulting methods (modeling, direct instruction, providing resources, or encouragement) and interaction styles (tell, sell, teach/advise, or encourage/support). Observe both the reactions of your partner and your own reactions, including positive and negative feelings and outcomes.

Conclusion

Deciding on your role as a consultant can be complicated and is specific to each situation. Three interrelated elements (intervention strategies, consulting methods, and interaction styles) largely influence your consulting role. In most situations, you will know from the beginning the desired educational outcomes and whose expertise is needed to achieve them. You will develop your role as you gather more data and speculate about strategies, methods, and interaction styles. We use the term *speculate* because these will, and should, change as your initial best guesses are confirmed or require revision.

You will use various strategies, methods, and interaction styles with different team members as you work on achieving specific outcomes for a particular student. You may sell an idea to a teacher with whom you have an established relationship at the same time you choose to support a student's father as he tries out the idea at home. Your choices concerning how to act in a certain situation may also change over time. You may decide upon a more directive approach during the initial phase of introducing a new program and move to a less directive role of encouraging the assistant in carrying out a new program. You significantly increase the effectiveness of your consultation when you consciously make choices about when and how to provide your services to team members.

Selected Readings

Dettmer, P., L. Thurston, and N. Dyck. 1993. *Consultation, collaboration and teamwork for students with special needs.* Boston: Allyn and Bacon.

This is an excellent textbook on collaborative consultation for special educators that discusses the basic skills needed by any professional consulting in the schools.

Dunn, W. 1991. Consultation as a process: How, when and why? In *School-based practice for related services,* edited by C. Royeen. Bethesda, MD: American Occupational Therapy Association.

Lesson 5 of this self-study series on school-based therapy focuses on the process of consultation in an education setting. Many case examples are presented to illustrate points and self-rating forms are included for successful communication. Discipline-specific application-to-practice sections for professionals in the fields of physical and occupational and speech-language pathology are provided.

Dunn, W., and P. Campbell. 1992. Designing pediatric service provision. In *Pediatric occupational therapy,* edited by W. Dunn, 139-160. Thorofare, NJ: Slack.

The authors, both occupational therapists, emphasize using a continuum of service models and provide excellent guidelines applicable to both occupational and physical therapy for choosing a service model to meet a student's needs.

Heron, T. and K. Harris. 1982. *The educational consultant.* Austin, TX: Pro-Ed.

These authors discuss the competencies that consultants should demonstrate, including technical expertise (pp. 38-39), effective communication skills (gaining acceptance, minimizing resistance, dealing with change, managing conflict), disseminating information (pp. 62-66), and coordinating skills (pp. 66-70).

Lippitt, G., and R. Lippitt. 1978. *The consulting process in action.* San Diego: University Associates.

This text contains an extensive discussion of roles based on their level of directiveness. The roles discussed, from least to most directive, are:

- objective observer/reflector: raises questions for reflection
- process counselor: observes the problem-solving process and raises issues about mirroring feedback
- fact finder: gathers data, stimulates thinking, and interprets alternatives
- identifier and linker: identifies alternatives and resources for client and helps assess consequences
- joint problem solver: offers alternatives and participates in decisions
- trainer educator: trains client
- informational expert: regards, links, and provides policy or practice decisions
- advocate: proposes guidelines, persuades, or directs in the problem-solving process

The book also includes a discussion about the criteria for role selection and the nature of the consulting contract.

Chapter 7 highlights:

- starting, maintaining, and concluding consulting relationships
- essential interpersonal skills needed for effective consultation
- typical consultation situations encountered in the four stages of consultation
- suggested activities to practice consulting skills

Chapter 7

The Stages of Consultation

All the world's a stage, and all the men and women merely players: They have their exits and their entrances; and one man in his time plays many parts.

Shakespeare. *As You Like It,* Act II, Scene VII

As with any relationship, consultation moves through predictable stages as the relationship progresses. We compare these stages to a successful, well-scripted play and use a theater analogy throughout this chapter to help you think about your role as a consulting therapist. We refer to each of four stages to discuss:

- Entry (Cast of Characters)
- Issue Definition (What's the Story?)
- Implementing Recommendations (Action!)
- Concluding (Curtain Call)

Each stage includes:

- Scripts—typical consultation situations that we have identified based on our experience and research
- A Look Behind the Scenes—the essential interpersonal skills needed to successfully complete each stage
- Dress Rehearsal—opportunities to practice some of the skills that have been identified in the text

Stage 1: Entry (Cast of Characters)

How you begin your consulting relationship will affect its ultimate outcome, so it is critical to make conscious decisions about your initial interactions with other team members. Typically, you will enter a classroom and become part of an existing team. First, recognize who decided that your service was needed because this will have a great impact on your reception. Did a teacher ask for specific help from a therapist? Did you suggest consultative services after the IEP team recommended occupational or physical therapy or did a parent request direct service? Perhaps a third party initiated the request; for instance, a special education supervisor may have decided that Mr. Schmenken needed assistance in vocational education for a student with physical disabilities.

Second, keep in mind that you have chosen consultation in order to improve a student's performance in school. In order to accomplish this task, you will also change some aspect of the school environment, classroom routines, or teacher instruction. Even when there is a strong indication that change will be positive, it still generates apprehension. The entrance of any newcomer, especially a consultant who may be viewed as an authority, may raise anxieties in team members about change, power, and dependency (Glidewell 1959). You should be prepared to deal with your team members' anxieties.

The following are typical situations encountered during the initial phases of educational consultations with suggestions for handling each situation. We have called these situations *scripts*.

Scripts for Stage 1: Entry

The First Meeting

As a consulting therapist, you have knowledge or skills that will supplement those of other team members. There is potential to create an unequal power relationship, with your team members feeling subordinate and apprehensive that you might usurp their positions or authority. Your team members may not even be aware of these feelings, but you should be alert to this possibility no matter how warm their welcome appears on the surface.

How can you deal with your team members' potential anxieties? Allow them to exert as much control as possible over the initial arrangements of your meetings. Let them decide when you will first meet, who will be there, and where the meeting will be held. Ask them when it would be most helpful to observe the student in the classroom or other school environment and try to meet their scheduling preferences. If your schedule is bound by school assignment or meeting conflicts, share this information with them. Expressing the desire to meet them more than halfway indicates your willingness to participate as an equal. You can also give your team members the opportunity to contribute to the agenda for your first meeting. Remember that your goal as a newcomer to the team is to support and reinforce your team members, never to usurp their authority.

Sizing Up One Another

Team members may challenge your knowledge, attitudes, philosophy, or goals, particularly if you are new to the school system or their team. On the other hand, team members might feel you are evaluating them to determine the cause of the student's problems and they may wind up feeling that they could not handle the situation on their own. This may be particularly troublesome for teachers and assistants who have many years of experience but not with the specific issue you are addressing. Awareness of these potential tensions can help you be prepared to deal with and avert possible problems (Gallesich 1982).

While you are "sizing each other up," be cautious of playing the expert who provides quick solutions to complex questions. Do not assume that the initial referral issue is the most serious one confronting the team. Before confiding a list of more important concerns, team members may need to develop a relationship with you and, very likely, you may need to learn more about the situation before you can offer helpful advice.

During the Entry stage, be patient and wait before jumping in with solutions. Concentrate on understanding team members' perspectives and convey the idea that you expect to learn from them as well as to assist with the student's needs. Before asking a team member to make changes, comment on something positive about the classroom or interactions with the student. By looking for positive attributes, listening to team members, and avoiding interruption with ideas of your own, you demonstrate respect for other team members' competencies. This respect may be particularly important for family members who might fear that not being a professional puts them at a disadvantage. We cannot overstate the importance of recognizing and reinforcing team members' effective strategies and interactions with students before asking them to make changes.

Owning Your Feelings

Entering into a new relationship can provoke anxiety for you also. You may be concerned about working in the school system, meeting the needs of new people, or being prepared to plan intervention for students with diagnoses or educational outcomes you have never before encountered. Look for positive ways to handle your own anxiety. You might talk to colleagues or a supervisor, role play, or mentally rehearse how to handle your new challenge.

Putting Personal Skills to Use

Team members often cite the personal qualities of a consultant as being more important than their professional competency (Schowengerdt, Fine, and Poggio 1976; Weissenburger, Fine, and Poggio 1982; West and Cannon 1988). One study of educators' satisfaction with consultation identified the top 10 interpersonal skills of the consultant:

1. practices in an ethical manner
2. maintains confidentiality
3. shows respect for consultee
4. knowledgeable
5. approachable
6. effective at establishing rapport
7. confident
8. trustworthy
9. understands the school system
10. good communicator

Knoff, McKenna, and Riser 1991

Interestingly, the least-favored attributes in this study included two that were expected (aggressive and authoritarian) and two that were surprising (colorful and funny). Apparently, the respondents (307 teachers) did not find humor or anecdotes helpful. On the contrary, we have found both attributes, if genuine and consistent with the consultant's personality, to be very helpful. Just be true to your nature.

What does this research suggest for your practice as a consulting therapist? Place a priority on establishing a positive relationship with all team members from the earliest interactions. Accept the teacher and all other team members as individuals, with strengths and needs. Show enough warmth and humanity to come across as a caring person. Act as an ethical, respectful, and knowledgeable therapist.

Behind the Scenes: Interpersonal Skills for Entry

Attitudes and Beliefs

It is essential to recognize the impact of your personal experiences and beliefs in creating expectations about how therapists should provide therapy or how teachers should organize their classrooms. You may believe that your primary mission is to treat students in the schools, especially when they have problems in traditional therapy domains, or you may feel that your job is to support teachers in their attempts to help students learn. Other personal missions therapists have shared with us include acting as a child advocate, change agent, assessor, resource, advisor, enabler, helper, and catalyst. Each role can positively or negatively influence your interactions with team members. As a consulting therapist, it is your responsibility to recognize the personal values governing your work in the schools and choose actions appropriate to each situation you encounter. Know how your actions are governed by your belief system and recognize the value judgments you subconsciously make. For instance, if a parent or teacher does not follow through with your suggestions, does that make the person a disorganized parent or teacher? Or does it indicate that you need to talk with the individual to find out why your suggestions are not working out? If you believe you are a student's advocate, what does that imply about your perception of the teacher's role? Can you both be advocates? What happens if you disagree on what will be helpful to achieve desired outcomes for the student? Does that make one person's ideas right and the other's wrong?

View of the World

Your tendency toward optimism or pessimism is important to recognize since it will affect how you measure your success as a consulting therapist. We all have external criteria from employers, colleagues, and consumers to judge our work performance, such as job evaluations, pay raises, recommendations, awards, and thank you letters. Each of us also carries an internal yardstick to measure our professional performance against a personal, usually private, standard. Consulting, because of its indirect nature, often does not provide clear indicators for us to judge our performance, especially if we are focused on seeing improvement in a student firsthand. Our personal view of the world may color our perceptions of how well we are doing with consulting. If a teacher likes two out of four recommendations, does that mean you are a good or ineffective therapist? Some consultants will be very pleased that the teacher liked at least half of the ideas. Others will think that they missed the mark on two of the four suggestions. You need to establish or refine your expectation regarding "success" as a consulting therapist compared to a direct service provider. Consulting therapists must learn to enjoy the process of helping others work effectively with students.

Dress Rehearsal: Entry

1. Introduce yourself in a way that conveys competence without being arrogant. First, write down your proposed introduction and then try it out on a trusted friend for feedback.

2. The next time you meet a new team member, comment on a positive aspect of the organization of the classroom or space, the person's interaction with students, or an instructional technique or resource that is new to you before discussing recommendations for change.

3. Visualize an interaction that you recently had with a new acquaintance with whom you find it difficult to work. Mentally replay the beginning of this relationship and visualize a more positive interaction and outcome.

Stage 2: Issue Definition (What's the Story?)

The ultimate goal of your consultation is to help a student achieve individualized goals and objectives. You judge your effectiveness by the improvement in the student's performance in school. As a consulting therapist, your method is to recommend intervention that someone else will carry out; that is, you translate your disciplinary expertise and experience to support other family and professional team members in their roles with a particular student.

You may be asked to adopt the role of a consultant, even though that may not be your job title. As you enter Stage 2, Issue Definition, remember that consultation is a:

> process based upon an equal relationship characterized by mutual trust and open communication, joint approaches to problem identification, the pooling of personal resources to identify and select strategies that will have some probability of solving the problem that has been identified, and shared responsibility in the implementation and evaluation of the program or strategy that has been initiated.
>
> Brown et al. 1979

If you perform any of these functions, you are acting as a consultant. Most school-based therapists are internal consultants who are considered staff or employees of the school system. Consultants are not always external experts who are brought into the schools to provide some advice on a specific issue. As Dick Darman, a former U.S. Budget Director, pointed out: "If it walks like a duck, quacks like a duck, and swims like a duck, then it's a duck!"

The first step in defining the issue is to assure the "buy-in" of all significant parties; in other words, ensure that everyone is aware of and in agreement about the student outcomes to be addressed. This task is often not as easy as it may appear. The presenting problem may not be the real issue at all, or one team member may have one perspective about the problem and another individual may have a completely different idea about why the student is not performing as expected. For example, a teacher may ask you for advice about positioning MyBinh, a student with multiple disabilities. However, what is really bothering the teacher is that it takes so much time for her assistant to feed MyBinh that the assistant is unable to help the other students at mealtime. If your suggestions for positioning MyBinh wind up taking even more time, it will be dropped very quickly. In another scenario, a teacher may think that a student's inability to attend during math class is a result of fatigue, while the mother may be convinced that her child is hungry. As the consulting therapist, your first priority is to assist all team members with agreeing on what the problem really is in order to identify possible solutions.

Scripts for Stage 2: Issue Definition

What's the Name of the Game?

As the consulting therapist, you need to identify and clarify the issue or need for change as perceived by the key stakeholders or team members. The ability to identify the student's needs as perceived by each team member is very important to the success of your consultation. One study found that the consultant's skill in eliciting information was predictive of her success in identifying the primary concern of team members (Bergan and Tombari 1976). Identification of the team members' concerns typically led to their eventual resolution, whereas a failure to identify the concerns more often resulted in a lack of success in developing and implementing an intervention plan.

Active listening, unobtrusive and sensitive questioning, and skillful dialogue will allow you to develop some hypotheses about the problems to be addressed. Ask your team members what they hope the student will accomplish in three months, six months, and by the end of the school year. You might ask, "If Johnny could feed himself, what would that action look like in six months?" or "How would we know Johnny has successfully mastered this outcome?" Find out how important these changes are compared to other priorities. Use paraphrasing and reflecting to confirm that you understand the needs and the goals as perceived by each team member.

Resisting the Quick Fix

Team members may want to change a student's behavior quickly, with a minimum of disruption or effort on their part. As a consulting therapist, you may be perceived as an authority who can offer quick solutions. Being viewed as the expert is quite seductive. However, being the revered expert is not the best role to adopt or to be assigned when your goal is to foster collaboration. All too often the team member inadvertently sets the expert up to fail because the expert is the expert and the team member is "only" the teacher (or assistant or family member). As you begin identifying the issues at hand, avoid quick, authoritative answers to early questions. In the initial stages, it is essential to listen, learn, and reflect on the other team members' concerns and the student's situation.

In addition, you should avoid appearing to be evasive or selfish with your knowledge. If team members really want to know what you think, share your hypothesis but emphasize that it is still a speculation until you gather more information. Many questions can be directed back to the teacher who probably has some tentative answers already or who may learn by hypothesizing and analyzing options. For instance, you may want to ask, "What possibilities occur to you?" "How have you dealt with this situation in the past?" Try to assist team members by focusing on the primary task of this stage, issue identification, and assure them that the team will begin to discuss solutions as soon as they have a shared understanding of the issues.

This issue identification stage requires a fine balance. In some serious or life-threatening situations, for example, students with fragile medical conditions, primitive reflexes, brittle bones, or fluctuating regulatory systems, you may need to give quick answers and deal with being so directive later. Also, if you perceive the teacher to be very frustrated, do not extend this exploratory period too long before suggesting a specific intervention with ample follow-up support. Just be aware that being too authoritative or jumping in with quick solutions may be detrimental to the development of a truly egalitarian relationship and you may need to address this issue after the immediate crises have been solved.

Tapping All Perspectives

When all parties participate in problem identification and decision making, the resulting intervention program is much more likely to be carried out. Team members have demonstrated a strong preference for consultation models in cases when the consultant shares the authority and decision making with them (Babcock and Pryzwansky 1983).

Your primary goal during Stage 2 (Issue Definition) is for all team members to have an equal representation in deciding how to meet the student's needs. Ask team members what they suggest or if anyone has had previous experience with regard to the issue and what strategies have worked in the past. Ask family and other team members about alternative ways that they can think of to meet the student's objectives. You should consider and respond to any suggested options. Acknowledge any new and creative ideas that this brainstorming brings up. Once all of the suggestions are on the table, the team can begin the process of prioritizing needs and developing goals and objectives.

Of course, you can contribute this valuable expertise only if you are present at the team meetings or have shared your issues and strategies with team members who can represent your viewpoints. Attendance may be difficult for some itinerant therapists. You may need administrative support so that you can be a contributing member of the team during this vital stage of issue identification and consensus-building. The ultimate success of school-based collaborative consultation may rest on this initial team processing.

Behind the Scenes: Interpersonal Skills for Issue Definition

Communication

Your ability to express your ideas, articulate concerns, and elicit information from others is vital to success throughout the consultation process, especially in Stage 2, when the goal is to establish common ground for agreeing on a student's needs and educational outcomes. Three skills in particular will help you with this task: active listening, using a common language, and reading verbal and nonverbal messages appropriately. Active listening is nonjudgmental and will help you accurately summarize and restate team members' ideas and perspectives. Using a common language means that you will eliminate as much professional jargon as possible. Some examples of incomprehensible jargon identified by teachers and family members include: *amphibian crawl, homolateral patterns, asymmetric tonic neck reflex, three jaw chuck,* and *vestibular* and *proprioceptive processing.* You probably can add your own favorites to the list. While jargon is a disciplinary shorthand, it sends a message of exclusivity when used with people who do not understand it. The third skill, reading messages appropriately, is especially important in terms of nonverbal cues and is not always easy to learn. However, when the sender's message is unclear, learn to ask for clarification. As illustrated in the following situation, you can save yourself ill will and valuable time.

Bruce, a therapist following up on his recommendations with Johnetta, a special educator, notices that she is not making eye contact with him and gives only short replies to his questions about how their program is going. He is puzzled because she has been enthusiastic in previous meetings. Fearing that his recommendations have hit a snag, Bruce asks if there is a problem. Johnetta blurts out, "Yes! I just received word that my son was in a car accident. He's okay but the car is badly damaged. I really need to leave right now." After expressing his sympathy, Bruce schedules another meeting. He easily could have misinterpreted Johnetta's verbal and nonverbal communication if he had not made the effort to clarify her implied message of avoidance.

Facilitation

The ability to influence and motivate others to plan together for a common goal are important skills for consulting therapists. In order to reach this high ground, you must make choices about problem-solving strategies, how to assist team members to come to consensus on recommendations, and when to vary your interaction style to promote team effort. Some of the qualities of good leaders which are particularly helpful for you to consider include being able to present a vision for programs and recruiting and motivating others to share their goals and mission (Mitchell and Tucker 1992).

Dress Rehearsal: Issue Definition

Practicing some of the communication strategies identified above will help you develop new skills and refine existing ones. The first activity suggested on the following page deals with understanding another's perspective. The second activity provides you with a method to review the use of jargon.

1. A narrative interview, or storytelling, is one way to understand other team members' perspectives when developing a plan (Hanft and Burke 1993). The following is an activity to assist you with understanding the power of listening to stories. Three people can participate in this activity and assume the roles of storyteller, listener, or reflecter of the interactions.

   Directions for the Storyteller. Think about something that your student does now that pleases you. Describe this "snapshot" (what the student did, who was there, what was happening, what led up to this event or action, and how the student felt).

   Directions for the Listener. Describe what happened in the storyteller's words. What does this story illustrate about the student? What facilitated this event or situation? What did you learn about the storyteller? What is the outcome of the story?

   Directions for the Reflecter. What did you notice about the communication and interaction between the listener and the storyteller?

   Try this same exercise a second time, with the storyteller describing something this same student will do within the next year. Describe what a future snapshot would look like (who would be there, what would happen, where and when the event would take place). This future snapshot indicates what the storyteller hopes the student will be able to learn and can lead to a discussion about specific educational outcomes for the student.

2. This exercise will help you determine the readability of your written reports and identify professional jargon by using the SMOG formula (Edmondson and Spell 1991). The SMOG formula assesses the reading or grade level needed to understand written material. This method is 68% accurate within 1½ grade levels. For this exercise you will need a report with at least 30 sentences in order to apply the SMOG formula. Mark off 10 sentences in each of three sections of the report—the beginning, the middle, and the end—and calculate the following:

   a. Count the number of words with three or more syllables, including repeats of any word. Pronounce numerals and abbreviations out loud to count syllables (for example, 16 = 2 syllables). Hyphenated words are considered one word. For example, the sentence "Shirley *demonstrates* a *radial digital* grasp on *materials* with the left hand" scores a 4. Each italicized word in this sample has three or more syllables.

   b. Find the nearest square root (in whole numbers, no fractions) of your total word count for the 30 sentences and add 3 to find the grade level. For example, the nearest square root for a total count of 85 words with 3 or more syllables would be 9; adding 3 would equal the twelfth grade level.

It is interesting to note that many professional or jargon words contain three or more syllables. Grading the readability of your reports can help you identify when you are using jargon and prompt you to think about appropriate alternatives. For example, the sentence in step (a) above could be rewritten in more understandable language for other team members without losing essential therapeutic information:

"Shirley uses her left hand to pick up toys, such as blocks, by holding them between her thumb and index and middle fingers (called a *radial digital grasp*)." By adding information about how Shirley's grasp pattern affects her performance in the classroom, you will make your report educationally relevant: "This type of grasp is immature for her age and makes it difficult for Shirley to pick up objects less than one inch wide since she does not use the tips of her fingers. As a result, she does not have the fine motor skills needed for coloring, making bead necklaces in art, or even turning the pages of a book one at a time."

Stage 3: Implementing Recommendations (Action!)

After identifying the student's functional problems and determining appropriate educational outcomes, you can begin planning how to achieve these goals. As a consulting therapist, your job is to motivate another team member to carry out your recommendations and provide support for doing so.

If the previous stages have gone smoothly, implementation may flow without difficulty as well. Once relationships have been established, problems have been identified and prioritized, and goals and objectives have been agreed upon, you can choose strategies to improve the student's performance and then carry them out.

Scripts for Stage 3: Implementing Recommendations

Ensuring Acceptance

Team members will be more likely to carry out the planned activity if:

- it is easy and convenient
- there is minimal disruption to their schedules
- the level of effort needed is "doable"
- they understand the rationale for any changes in how they work with students
- the recommended activities are congruent with their existing curricula

Using your knowledge of the classroom will help you design activities that can be integrated into the daily schedule. For example, if you want to improve a student's hand grip, try modifying existing activities, such as handwriting drills or art projects. If you must make changes in equipment or class routines, first try small modifications. If you are still not satisfied with the student's progress, talk with team members about why other modifications are needed or why you are suggesting a procedure that appears inconvenient to them. Remember, what's "old hat" to you may be radically different to a teacher or family member. Try to enlist support from the team members before introducing what they may view as radically new equipment or different procedures. Always stay focused on strategies that are educationally relevant.

Supporting Change

As a consulting therapist, you will be expected to suggest new ideas and be the final decision maker about interventions that are part of your disciplinary expertise. After you have facilitated everyone's input, carefully consider it and add your own recommendations. You can be recognized for your expertise without having to be the expert. Make sure that your recommendations match the level of comfort and expertise of your team members.

If your recommendations represent changes in school routines, schedules, equipment, materials, or interactions with the student, you must consider how to support other team members so they will feel comfortable with the change. You might want to reconsider your strategies, methods, and interaction styles as discussed in chapter 6. As team members begin to implement the jointly agreed-upon activities, you should be prepared to quickly assist if any problems arise. Your team members may expect to spend time and effort developing an intervention plan with you during Stages 1 and 2, but they may not realize how much effort is required to communicate productively during implementation. You may need to be the person who ensures that this communication occurs.

Ongoing Communication

When finalizing plans for carrying out agreed-upon tasks, build in a schedule for ongoing feedback. This is a time when you should sensitively utilize your own professional expertise to monitor, redesign, and evaluate activities as necessary to meet the student's needs. You must make sure you know how the team's plans are being carried out and if something needs to change. Depending on your schedule and the preferences of your team members, this feedback might include direct interactions with the student in the class or at home, written notes or journals shared among all team members, or scheduled telephone calls. In some cases, you may find yourself the nucleus of a communication network involving the student, the family, classroom personnel, and other specialists. This networking is time-consuming but crucial to the success of the student's progress. If you find that a problem exists, be prepared to take quick action. If a major problem with your intervention plan arises, you may need to call the whole team back together or spend some time in the classroom trying out alternatives until everyone is satisfied. In other cases, your plan might need only minor modifications.

Finally, the consulting therapist should share positive impressions about what is working and encourage everyone to celebrate each milestone as it is accomplished. Shared celebrations go a long way in developing positive relationships and minimizing conflicts.

Behind the Scenes: Interpersonal Skills for Implementing Recommendations

Negotiation

The most important interpersonal skill for Stage 3 (and other stages as well) is the ability to negotiate; that is, reconcile different perspectives, coordinate strategies, recognize and defuse turf battles, and manage conflict as you implement the consulting plan. We have devoted chapter 9 to identifying typical consultation conflicts that arise in each of the four stages and offer specific strategies for conflict resolution.

Dress Rehearsal: Implementing Recommendations

The following suggestions focus on scheduling follow-up observations, trying alternative communication strategies, and celebrating successes.

1. Look over your school calendar. Schedule time for 20-minute follow-up observations and communication sessions with key team members for each of your students. Only you know how often you need to check in with a given student and a specific teacher, but chances are these follow-up observations will not occur if you do not plan them.

2. Choose three students for whom you want to improve follow-up sessions. Consider follow-up models that you want to try out or refine, such as telephone calls, written notes, notebooks, in-person contacts, photos and drawings, or other mechanisms you think of that will enhance communication among all team members. Contact the key team members for each of these three students and choose the type of follow-up that best meets all of your needs. Try out the techniques for one month and then review the results.

3. While you have your calendar out, check to see which holidays, inservices, or planning times are coming up during the next three months. Look for a time to celebrate your combined successes. You may plan to celebrate with those team members who have made the most progress or with team members with whom you want to develop better relationships. Ask them to have lunch with you on inservice days and focus on what has been going well and the progress that the student has made.

Stage 4: Concluding (Curtain Call)

When students have achieved their specified outcomes, it is time to close that specific objective or conclude your consultation entirely. You and your team members may decide to work on other problems affecting a student's educational performance and begin another cycle of planning and implementation or you may decide to conclude your consultation. Ending consultative relationships positively is your final responsibility in the process and is the one act that is typically left out of the entire play.

The best way to deal with concluding your services is to plan for it well in advance. At the initial IEP meeting there should be discussion about how long you expect the team will need your consultative services. This discussion emphasizes that consultation is expected to be a time-limited relationship, not an open-ended service option that continues for years. As soon as you foresee that your services will no longer be needed, you should share this information with your team members, preferably in a meeting. You can address any team members' concerns, including those of the family, at this time as well as during your final consultations. As you reduce your presence in the classroom, be sure to transfer any remaining responsibilities to other team members as needed.

Successful conclusion of this last stage is critical to the accomplishments of student outcomes, to the satisfaction of team members, and to the ultimate perception team members have of the value of the consultation model. If a team member feels the conclusion has been poorly undertaken, that the student has been dropped prematurely, or that the team is being abandoned by the therapist, future successful consultation relationships are compromised. However, if everyone is prepared and satisfied with the conclusion, the benefits of collaborative consultation will make themselves known to all parties of the consultative relationship. Establishing a history of successful consultation supports the appropriate use of this intervention method.

Scripts for Stage 4: Concluding

Evaluation

An intervention plan is not complete until you evaluate the results of your efforts. From the onset, you need to identify how you, the student, the family, and the educational team will know if the plan is working. To keep informed about progress, you need to decide what data needs to be collected, by whom, how, and how often. When and how will you reconvene to determine if everything is going according to plan and the student is retaining the progress that has been made?

Acknowledging Feelings

Careful consideration of how this leave-taking is going to affect you, the student, family members, and the other staff with whom you have been working will ease this transition. All transitions involve some emotions. We discuss how to deal with potentially negative emotions in chapter 9. These emotions may include sadness, relief, exhilaration, or even anger. You need to anticipate and deal with your own and your team members' feelings appropriately so that you can end this consultative relationship on a positive note.

Judging Success

When you provide direct therapy, you decide if you have done a good job by judging the student's progress. When you consult, you need to develop another way to judge professional performance. You will still judge success based on the student's accomplishments, but you will also want to know how well you did as a consulting therapist.

Do not judge yourself solely on the basis of your team members' satisfaction with your services. If you have been successful at achieving a collaborative relationship, they may not even be aware of how hard and how well you have worked. Consider what went well, why, and what you wish you had done differently. You might arrange a team get-together for everyone to discuss "what-ifs" or you could meet with significant players on an individual basis to give you feedback about your consultation. A reproducible self-evaluation form is included on page 150.

Celebration

To end the consultative relationship on a positive note, consider arranging a party or other celebration to give everyone, including the student, a chance to part with a sense of a job well done.

Behind the Scenes: Interpersonal Skills for Concluding

Political savvy

Political savvy in this context refers to a collection of interrelated skills to help you analyze past, present, and future consulting situations and relationships in order to make changes in your current ones. We believe it is important to review your student-specific consultation as well as the larger picture of the consultation services you provide. Do you know who to go to for support; that is, who are the school decision- and policymakers? Can you plan and carry out a course of action when needed? Whether you end a relationship with a team member because a student's objective has been achieved or begin work on developing a plan to address a new objective, it is important to look at what has transpired and think about any changes you would like to make in future interactions.

Sometimes you may discover that there is a discrepancy between the personal mission you have for yourself as a consulting therapist and other team members' expectations of what they hope to accomplish by working with students in the schools. Your political savvy can guide you to assess with whom to talk and what to do next. Knowledge of federal and state special education laws and regulations is also important to help you evaluate the appropriateness of your consulting services. A principal, for instance, may give you her interpretation of what the Federal law says about providing for related services or present district policy as if it were law. For example, therapists have been told erroneously by school administrators that they can work only with students with severe physical involvement or that all services for students with learning disabilities must be provided through a consultation model.

Dress Rehearsal: Concluding

Klein and Kontos (1993) developed a consultant skills inventory that we have modified to serve as a vehicle for you to monitor your current performance as a consultant on a regular basis. (Please see page 150 of the appendix for the reproducible skills inventory.) You will not excel at every skill on this self-evaluation, but over time, completing such a checklist regularly will give you a fairly accurate portrait of your strengths and areas in which you need to improve your skills. We recommend that you complete the checklist fairly frequently. Today, choose a student and situation about which you feel very competent and look back over your related interactions during the last month. For each item, rate your own skill level according to the scale given.

Conclusion

Consultation is an interactive process with specific stages. The skillful therapist recognizes this cycle and considers how and when to move the consultation through the stages of entry, issue definition, implementing recommendations, and conclusion. While team members are always considered partners in the consultative relationship, the therapist must take the initiative to "facilitate and examine the process, and change its course if the process does not seem to be working" (Bundy 1991, p. 325). This is accomplished by selecting a variety of intervention strategies, consulting methods, and interaction styles to effectively assist team members to meet student needs, enabling them to function and learn in the school environment.

Selected Readings

Bundy, A. 1991. Consultation and sensory integration theory. In *Sensory integration: Theory and practice,* edited by A. Fisher, E. Murray, and A. Bundy, 317-32. Philadelphia: F. A. Davis.

In this text, consultation is defined and illustrated with case examples of how to apply sensory integration principles to promote a better "fit" between the school and home environments (human and nonhuman) and the child. The problems and possible solutions to the four stages of consultation are discussed: formulating expectations, establishing a partnership, planning strategies, and implementing/assessing the plan.

Jaffee, E., and C. Epstein. 1993. The process of consultation. In *Occupational therapy consultation,* edited by E. Jaffee and C. Epstein. St. Louis: Mosby.

The authors, both occupational therapists, present an interesting and comprehensive discussion of the stages of consultation that they call *cycles* (pp. 135-166). This text is an excellent resource for consultants who want to learn more details about the process of consultation, especially what the authors refer to as the four Ps of consultation: power, politics, problems, and pitfalls. The cycles they describe are:

- entry into the system
- negotiation of contract
- diagnostic analysis leading to problem identification
- goal setting and planning through establishment of trust
- maintenance phase of intervention and feedback
- evaluation
- termination
- possible renegotiation of contract

Lippitt, G., and R. Lippitt. 1978. *The consulting process in action.* San Diego: University Associates.

This text describes six phases of consultation and the focuses of each phase.

- Phase I: Contact and Entry
- Phase II: Formulating a Contract and Establishing a Helping Relationship
- Phase III: Problem Identification and Diagnostic Evaluation
- Phase IV: Goal Setting and Planning
- Phase V. Taking Action and Cycling Feedback
- Phase VI: Contract Completion: Continuity, Support, Termination

Chapter 8 describes the five personal and institutional variables that both support and challenge effective consultation:

- time demands
- administrative support
- team members' attitudes
- knowledge of consultation
- professional expertise/ experience

Chapter 8

Supports for and Challenges to Successful Consultation

Once upon a time there was a grasshopper who decided to consult a wise old owl about his suffering through many cold winters. The owl listened patiently to the grasshopper's misery and offered this simple advice: "Simply turn yourself into a cricket and hibernate during the winter." After discovering that this important knowledge could not be transformed into action, the grasshopper returned to the owl and asked how he could perform this metamorphosis. The owl replied curtly, "Look, I gave you the principle. It's up to you to work out the details!"

Warren Bennis, quoted in Apter 1994

The comment from Warren Bennis, an expert on leadership and organizational development, that introduces this chapter is an apt reminder that identifying your goals does not ensure that their accomplishment will be effortless. Deciding to expand your role as a consulting therapist in schools and developing the necessary skills for this role do not guarantee your success. The following five personal and institutional variables can have either a positive or negative impact on your ability to consult effectively:

- time demands
- administrative support
- team members' attitudes and expectations
- knowledge and skills for consultation
- professional expertise/experience

Time

Lack of time is one of the most daunting barriers to providing effective consultation in the schools (Idol-Maestas and Ritter 1985; Johnson, Pugach, and Hammittee 1988; Speece and Mandell 1980; McGlothlin and Kelly 1982). As discussed in chapter 1, one of the prevailing myths regarding consultation is that therapists can double or triple their case loads by using this service model.

Consultation is an indirect way to enhance student performance by working with teachers, teaching assistants, other specialists, family members, and students. It is time-consuming to talk with all these team members, observe students in school settings, share perspectives and observations, identify common educational outcomes, and plan intervention. All of these tasks must be completed before your recommendations can even be implemented. Once you begin implementation, you must also evaluate how well your program or interventions are working—another critical time-consuming task.

Ironically, even arranging when and where to meet and talk with team members requires time. Therapists are not alone in bemoaning the lack of time available for collaboration. Many special education teachers and classroom teachers report that they simply do not have enough time within their school day to collaborate (Stainback and Stainback 1985; Idol-Maestas 1983). Moreover, special educators are often expected to consult with general education teachers and often use their own planning time to work in these meetings (Neel 1981).

Strategies for Finding Time to Consult

Educators have identified several important ways to structure time for collaborating with one another (Dettmer, Thurston, and Dyck 1993). Therapists may also find these strategies helpful.

Create "release time" by arranging for peer tutors, volunteers, administrators, student teachers, or substitutes to free up classroom teachers for collaboration.

Team teach with colleagues to give one another time to talk with consultants.

Schedule staff meeting time at periodic intervals without students present; for example, every fourth Wednesday after students leave or one day per marking period.

Meet during the school day, such as before and after school, at lunch, or during periods when students are in music or PE classes.

Plan special events at regular intervals, such as assemblies, films, guest speaker visits, and plays, to free up some teachers for collaboration.

Hire a permanent rotating substitute, possibly with funds donated from local business groups or other sources. In some school districts, principals and other administrators teach a class at specific times to free teachers for collaboration.

Therapists also need to manage their time and find creative ways to meet with team members. In addition, they need to find time to observe and work with students in classrooms and other environments in which students are expected to learn and perform, such as playgrounds, lunch rooms, physical education classes, and field trips. The following are some recommended strategies:

Rotate school visits and vary schedules so you are not always in the same school at the same time on the same days. This process will create greater opportunities for you to see students in different activities during the school day. Schedule the beginning or end of the day in the school at which you have the most students so you can talk with their teachers before or after school.

Plan and lead an activity for the entire class with the teacher to give you an opportunity to observe particular students. Demonstrate an activity that the teacher can do again at another time when you will not be there.

Try out recommended interventions first so the teacher can observe what you do. This strategy allows you to determine trouble spots and modify the intervention immediately.

Use block scheduling to allow for extended time in the classroom beyond the traditional 30 to 45 minutes allocated for individual therapy (Benson 1993; Rainforth, York, and MacDonald 1992). Therapy periods for several students are combined in a block of time once per week or every other week, enabling the therapist to work with these students in a greater variety of activities.

Use written communication whenever possible. Keep a notebook in the classroom that is divided into sections by the students you work with for writing comments to teachers and parents. One school district provides therapists with carbonless paper to jot notes to teachers and to send home while also keeping a copy for themselves. Send an information sheet to a teacher describing what you will be working on or hope to observe before you visit the classroom. One mother in a rural area gave her son's therapist stamped and addressed postcards to send back to her with weekly feedback.

Administrative and Family Support

Educators and therapists have reported that lack of administrative support is another major barrier to implementing a successful consultation program (Clark and Porsch 1993; Idol-Maestas and Ritter 1985). As educators have noted:

> Administrators must assume responsibility for scheduling the time needed by consultants and consultees to collaborate. If they lend their authority to this endeavor, school personnel will be more willing to brainstorm ways of getting together.
>
> Dettmer, Thurston, and Dyck 1993

Enlisting administrative support. Needless to say, it is extremely important to enlist the support of school administrators, occupational and physical therapy supervisors, teacher supervisors, principals, and special education directors, for your consultation activities before making major changes in how you provide therapy to students. Apter (1994) identifies five important lessons for guiding systems change in early intervention that we have adapted for you to consider when initiating or expanding consultation in the schools. These are discussed below.

Everyone involved must be convinced that consultation is rational and that they will gain from these services. Strive to understand the perspective of all stakeholder groups—school administrators and supervisors, teachers, families, students, and other specialists. Also consider how individual reactions to consultation; for instance, "Great! I can get help right in my classroom," or "Uh oh, my class routine will be disturbed."

Everyone involved must be educated to change expectations about how therapy services are delivered and develop commitment to new ways. Do not assume that stakeholders understand what consultation is. They may already have a conceptualization of consultation that does not match yours. Your state special education regulations may already define consultation. In our experience, therapists often have very different ideas about what consultative services are and how they should be provided in the schools.

Teachers and therapists can be forced to change by school administrators or peer pressure, but this approach also carries negative consequences. Enlist the support of school administrators who are responsible for related services as well as general and special education, but do not rely on administrative edict to change attitudes. Remember that families are not employees of the school system and have different concerns than educators and therapists.

Never fail to respect and understand the resisters and the positive nature of their resistance (Klein 1976; Marris 1986). Listen to those teachers, therapists, and family members who resist change with regard to how therapists provide services since it may signal loss from their perspective. They may be pointing out aspects of your therapy program that are important to keep. Too much resistance indicates a need for more planning and discussion.

Leadership is necessary at every level of planning for success in implementing expanding consultative therapy services. Administrative support is critical, but you must also assume a leadership role and be able to articulate your vision of how consultation will enhance students' performance in school. All physical and occupational therapists should work together to provide similar services. It is very difficult to be the lone therapist consulting in the classroom when everyone else utilizes a different model.

Table 8.1 offers eight guidelines for designing and implementing consulting therapy services that incorporate the five lessons above. While you may be successful consulting with some teachers on your own initiative, we highly recommend that you work with your occupational and physical therapy colleagues to develop a consultation model as a group or department. This process ensures uniformity throughout your school district.

Keep in mind that families are an important stakeholder group for enlisting support from the beginning. Many parents believe the "more is better" principle, based on their experience receiving occupational and physical therapy from hospital-based or private clinicians. Some parents believe, and may have experienced, that consultation means their children will receive less service than what they need. Consultation is then viewed as a deterrent to achieving desired educational outcomes. We highly recommend that you consider how to address family concerns and solicit their involvement as you develop, implement, and critique your consultation services.

Table 8.1
Gaining Support for School-Based Consultation

Action Step	Why	Examples
1. Read literature and interview other therapists and educators.	To clarify your role as a consulting therapist, to understand the difference between consultation and direct service, and to develop a personal vision for providing consultation in the schools.	Read therapy and education literature on consultation. Explore what the professional literature says about consultation. To learn about the experiences of others, interview therapists and educators who consult. Choose role models of excellence. Ask each for their three most important tips.
2. Develop a description of consultation services.	Formulate why and how consultation can benefit students in your school district as a basis for developing a formal plan.	Develop a one-page fact sheet explaining the benefits of occupational and physical therapy services in the schools, including different service models, to highlight the different forms of consultation that can be provided.
3. Meet with school administrators and supervisors.	It is essential that you enlist support from the decision makers in your setting. Do not proceed without their support.	Present your data, fact sheets, research studies (see table 8.3), and other resources that highlight consultation to principals, OT and PT supervisors, education supervisors, and special education directors.
4. Solicit support and reactions from stakeholders.	Talk with the people who will be most affected by how you deliver your therapy services, including general and special educators, other school therapists, family members, and students.	Form an advisory committee with stakeholders to review your plan and help you identify challenges and supports.
5. Prepare a plan for implementing consultation services.	Provide a written plan for stakeholders, including administrators, to consider. Use clear language and avoid professional jargon.	Topics to address: benefits of OT/PT consultation, teacher and therapist inservice needs and strategies for training, description of consultation with examples, suggestions for when and how to collaborate with teachers and work with students, how to solicit parental support and document consultation on IEPs.

Table 8.1 (continued)

Action Step	Why	Examples
6. Revise and finalize plan.	Go back to stakeholders, including decision makers, and show them your developing plan to seek continued support.	Present plan at inservice sessions and staff meetings and present various consultation scenarios for students of different ages and learning needs. Show how consultation services would help address desired student outcomes. Include information in memos and newsletters.
7. Implement the plan in stages.	Do not try to make dramatic revisions in service delivery for every student all at once.	Work out a schedule for implementation, starting with educators and parents who are the most receptive.
8. Solicit feedback and revise your plan.	Critique your efforts. Identify challenges that need to be addressed and successes that can be expanded.	Ask for feedback from stakeholders and therapists via surveys, focus groups, and personal interviews. Ask a school official to solicit comments from teachers and family members. Share information and recommendations for revisions with administrators and stakeholders.

Attitudes and Expectations

Team members may expect consulting therapists to work miracles to resolve a student's functional problems. Educators and parents often hope that someone else holds the key to positive change. These feelings are often transferred to therapists when parenting and teaching strategies have not produced the desired results in a student's learning and behavior. A closely related expectation is that the consulting therapist will be an expert and will know just what to do about the student's difficulties. When therapists do not have all or any answers, raise additional concerns based on their professional viewpoints, or suggest an intervention that appears to make no sense, team members may feel resentful about the time and energy they have put into talking with the therapist without obtaining results.

Team members may also have very specific ideas about how therapists should work with students. Some teachers may want therapists to take students out of their classroom, giving them a break from the sole responsibility for managing difficult behavior. Others expect that therapists will work solely in the classroom, helping them with daily routines and activities.

Addressing expectations

Suggesting interventions that make sense to other team members is dependent on your ability to see situations from their perspectives. Review the points raised in chapter 4 regarding human resources. What are other team members trying to accomplish? How can you help them change the student's behavior and learning?

What experiences have they had working with children who have abilities and difficulties similar to the student you are consulting with them about? Just as important, have they had any experiences with physical or occupational therapy? If so, these prior experiences will probably positively and negatively influence their expectations for how you should provide services. If all of the teacher's experience has been with direct service, you will need to carefully plan how to offer consultation. One therapist related her delight in finding out that her teacher had previous experience with a consulting therapist until she heard how awful the experience was. It took more than six months of careful interaction before the teacher accepted that this therapist really was different from the previous one. We recommend six strategies for fitting in the schools as a consulting therapist:

Work as an equal, not an authority. Be a team member with expertise in specific areas of student performance. Avoid acting as a supervisor, expert, or evaluator. Recognize and support teacher abilities and positive attributes about classroom activities. Look for resources about common areas of interest. Share your success in terms of "we"; for example, "You should see the progress Lin made when Mrs. Anderson and I found the right way to keep her sitting up!"

Participate in school routines. Do not hold yourself above performing some daily classroom duties and routines. One therapist who worked with preschoolers told her teammates she refused to change diapers because her intervention was too important to interrupt, so she would bring the child to the classroom aide for changing. Needless to say, she not only lost time but much goodwill by refusing to help out during her time in the classroom. Another therapist relates a humorous story about taking over a reading group during a classroom emergency. She was asked to direct a workbook activity that involved matching beginning sounds with a picture of the object. Seeing a chicken but no corresponding "ch," she instructed the students to write in the correct response. A little voice piped up from the back of the room that the chicken was a hen and matched the "h" on the worksheet. The classroom teacher appreciated this therapist's willingness to help out and went out of her way to solicit the therapist's input whenever she could.

Nurture relationships with teachers and other team members. Whenever possible, spend time with team members during the school day. One expert in school practice recommends socializing with teachers in the office, photocopy room, and faculty lounge. Be careful that you do not limit your support group to other therapists or you may wind up "teamless," especially if you serve a number of schools. Some therapists mistakenly believe that only members of their particular discipline can be part of their support group. In our experience, we have found numerous colleagues who shared many of our concerns and values. Itinerant therapists know how important it is to develop ongoing relationships with colleagues whenever they can.

Expect to learn from others and acknowledge when you do. Give others credit for their knowledge as well as their experience. A teacher's aide may not have a college degree, but her 15 years of experience working in the classroom with students who have multiple disabilities is worth its weight in gold. As a therapist working in schools, there is much to learn about the educational system. Teacher certification, special educators' training, reading curriculums, cooperative learning groups, portfolio assessments, transition to work programs, and kindergarten screenings may be parts of the school setting that are unfamiliar to therapists. Teachers for the hearing and visually impaired, school psychologists, speech-language pathologists, and other school specialists have unique strategies and "tricks" just as you do. In addition, family members can provide vital information about their child's interests and abilities that you would never have the opportunity to learn.

Incorporate principles of adult learning as you assist others in implementing your recommendations. Adult learners, when presented with new information, integrate the material by relating it to what they already know. Your interactions with team members should reinforce four basic principles of adult learning:

- Learning, yours and theirs, is continuous.
- Instructional methods must accommodate diverse learning styles, so use a multitude of strategies, including videos, printed materials, and demonstrations.
- Adults have personal agendas and a bank of previous experiences upon which to build.
- Adults learn new material by applying it to their own situations and trying it out.

(Gordon, Zemke, and Jones 1981; Merriam and Cunningham 1989)

Ask for feedback about your consultation. Evaluate how well you:

- developed your plan for consultation (see page 150 of the appendix for a self-rating form)
- suggested practical interventions that address educational outcomes and teacher/family concerns
- varied your intervention strategies, methods for translating knowledge to other adults, and interaction style to fit the needs of the other team members (see chapter 6)

Professional Expertise and Experience

In addition to knowledge about consultation, therapists must have specialized skills and knowledge to contribute to the team's task of enhancing the student's learning. Chapter 2 outlines important therapeutic domains and related educational outcomes that therapists must be skillful in addressing in the schools. The challenge is to contribute these skills and knowledge in a way that is meaningful to educators and other team members; that is, translate disciplinary expertise to assist other team members as they work with and care for students with special learning needs. This is the essence of effective school-based consultation.

Sometimes disciplinary expertise goes awry, resulting in turf battles and professional one-upmanship about whose service is most important. This can happen between physical and occupational therapists or between therapists and educators or other family members. When therapists do not feel respected or that their services are valued, it is easy to become overprotective about what programs and strategies they consider to be their own.

Since therapists, educators, and families have different experiences and knowledge, they may have significant problems communicating with one another, resulting in a lack of credibility for one another's suggestions and recommendations. This situation happens even between special and general educators who at least share a common goal of teaching children in schools (Johnson, Pugach, and Hammittee 1988).

Often therapists and educators use different terms to describe or categorize the same behavior. While therapists describe a student with poor coordination and reading problems as having a sensory integration disorder with dyspraxia, educators talk about a specific learning disability or dyslexia. A therapist may identify a neurological cause for behavior problems whereas a teacher points to a lack of motivation or interest for the subject area. The vignette at the beginning of chapter 2 (page 15) captures the difficulty that therapists encounter when using jargon with teachers as well as parents. In this instance, the parent explains to the therapist that in her family an RUE (right upper extremity) is called an ARM.

Strategies for Developing and Sharing Professional Expertise

We believe professional diversity is to be recognized and applauded for its positive impact on developing creative and unique ways to help students learn and perform in the school or other environment. The following strategies encourage therapists to share their expertise and learn from families and other specialists.

Disseminate successful school-based strategies and programs through presentations at regional, state, and national conferences and in professional publications of both therapy and education fields. Aim for cross-dissemination of ideas. Read and publish articles in educational journals such as *Topics in Early Childhood Special Education, Teaching Exceptional Children, Journal of Early Intervention, Remedial and Special Education, Exceptional Children, Child Development,* and *Phi Beta Kappa.*

Keep current in your own professional field. Join your professional association. Attend at least one professional seminar or workshop per year. Present an inservice for interdisciplinary colleagues about what you learned at a workshop and suggest ways to implement new strategies in the schools. Read a journal article every month. Find out what issues are emerging and stay abreast of recommended practices in your profession.

Start an information exchange over a brown bag lunch or breakfast once per month to review current journal articles and books related to school-system practice and, in particular, consultation. Make the focus of these exchanges interdisciplinary. Select a topic in advance and ask everyone to bring and discuss a great article from their discipline that relates to the topic. Bring copies of the articles for everyone. Write up all comments and share them with colleagues in other schools or districts.

Learn to communicate professional expertise without jargon. Ask a trusted colleague to give you a signal every time you use professional jargon. At staff or team meetings, give one person the responsibility to "blow the whistle" on anyone who uses terms, abbreviations, or acronyms that are unique to a particular field and may not be understood by all. Critique your reports by circling all words with two or more syllables (most often the professional terms). Invite parents to submit their "favorite" words that they often hear from professionals to an interdisciplinary jargon contest and suggest understandable substitutions. You may be surprised at the words that some families find difficult to understand or offensive. One family member objected to the use of the term *sibling* because her children were called brothers and sisters until her child with disabilities was born. Then professionals referred to them as siblings. Another mother disliked the term *parent involvement* because therapists cannot judge how involved parents are with their children on the basis of what they see in school or therapy sessions.

Recognize that more than one discipline can address a student's developmental needs and educational outcomes. The crucial element is to first identify what the student needs to learn, then decide who can "make it so" (Jean-Luc Picard, *Star Trek: The Next Generation*). When discussion begins about whether a student needs physical or occupational therapy before there is any agreement on educational outcomes, it is easy to feel displaced when occupational or physical therapy is not identified as a needed service on the IEP. For example, a student whose educational outcome is to move in and out of his seat independently in class can benefit from physical or occupational therapy, special education, or a combination of these services. Table 8.2 offers a framework for looking at the similarities and differences in how each of these disciplines provides intervention, using motor skills for young children as an example.

Conduct inservices and seminars for educators, families, and other team members based on a needs assessment they complete. Follow up to find out how team members used the information you presented. After attending a conference or workshop or reading a particularly helpful article, write and circulate a short summary and make your materials and notes available for review (Dettmer, Thurston, and Dyck 1993).

Table 8.2
Role of Occupational and Physical Therapists and Special Educators in Developing Motor Skills in Children

Area of Expertise	Occupational Therapy	Physical Therapy	Special Education
Sensorimotor development	Sensory and motor processing *Specialty: Influence of sensory input on adaptive behavior and functional motor skills*	Sensory and motor processing *Specialty: posture, balance, and quality of movement*	Impact of sensory impairments on learning
Neuromuscular function	Evaluate muscle tone, reflexes, and range of motion of legs, arms, and trunk and how they influence self-care, play, and motor skills *Specialty: arm and hand function*	Evaluate muscle tone, reflexes, and range of motion of legs, arms, and trunk and how they influence self-care, play, and motor skills *Specialty: mobility and stability of back, hips, legs*	Impact on movement, self-care, and play in school, home, and child-care settings
Motor development	Gross and fine motor skills and impact of neurological status on development *Specialty: fine motor, eye-hand coordination, visual-motor skills*	Gross and fine motor skills and impact of neurological status on development *Specialty: gross motor skills, balance and equilibrium, coordination*	Gross and fine motor skills
Adaptive equipment	Evaluation and recommendation for positioning equipment based on functional need; for example, corner chair, wheelchair, prone stander *Specialty: making hand splints; adapting feeding utensils, toys, and environment*	Evaluation and recommendation for positioning equipment to prevent structural deformity; for example, corner chair, wheelchair, prone stander *Specialty: training to use leg braces, orthotics*	Use of positioning equipment in school, home, child-care, and play environments
Functional movement	Use of body for play, communication, and self-care *Specialty: feeding, play, toileting, and dressing*	Mobility and walking *Specialty: locomotion, especially walking, body mechanics, and energy conservation*	Impact of movement on learning

Source: Adapted with permission from an early intervention workshop presented by B. Hanft, K. Sippel, and J. Pokorni on May 17-19, 1994, in Atlanta, Georgia.

Knowledge of Consultation

In order to consult effectively, therapists must possess certain skills and knowledge about the consulting process. This expertise includes knowledge of providing educationally relevant therapy in the schools and the ability to present a wide range of alternative interventions to assist team members. You should understand the stages of the consulting process (chapter 7) as well as how to use various methods to assist others with carrying out your recommendations and when to vary your interaction style (chapter 6). In addition, chapter 7 identifies the following interpersonal variables that influence your ability to develop and maintain successful consulting relationships with educators, family members, and other team members:

- attitudes and beliefs about the role of a consultant
- your view of the world and sense of humor
- recognition of how to obtain professional gratification by working indirectly to assist students
- communication and negotiation skills
- "political savvy" or the ability to analyze a situation and solicit support from decision makers

Familiarity with the literature regarding the effectiveness of school-based consultation can also provide you with data for soliciting support from administrators and other stakeholders. Table 8.3 summarizes five school-based studies that look at the effectiveness of occupational and physical therapy using a consultation model. In addition, three conclusions drawn from the special education and school psychology literature on the benefits of consultation are important for therapists to consider with regard to their own consultation (Idol, Nevin, and Paolucci-Whitcomb 1994; Medway and Updyke 1985):

1. Students with special education needs have benefitted from collaborative consultation between special and general educators. Students also benefit from collaboration between therapists and special/general educators.

2. Education personnel have learned the necessary skills and knowledge for collaborating with one another. Therapists can also acquire these skills.

3. Consultation has resulted in changes in student achievement (behavior, reading, math, and language), the service system (more appropriate referrals, inclusion in general education classes), and the adults involved in consulting relationships (enhanced teaching strategies, increased confidence, improved communication). Therapists can effect similar student, system, and adult changes.

Table 8.3
Occupational and Physical Therapy Studies of Consultation

Source	Aspect of Consultation Addressed	Description	Outcome
Campbell, McInerney, and Cooper (1984)	Incorporating therapy techniques with functional activities in an education setting	Therapists taught other team members to facilitate reaching for three students with severe disabilities	Students' movement increased when given greater opportunity to practice

Table 8.3 (continued)

Source	Aspect of Consultation Addressed	Description	Outcome
Giangreco (1986)	Effectiveness of direct versus integrated therapy; teacher provides therapeutic activities prior to switch training instruction	Single-subject reversal design for facilitating switch-control skills for a 13-year-old girl with multiple disabilities	Significant increase in the student's ability to activate the switch during integrated therapy phases
Cole et al. (1989)	Comparison of effects of in-class and out-of-class therapy on gross and fine motor performance; also surveyed teacher preferences for models	61 preschool children (28 with motor delays and 33 without) were randomly assigned to either therapy group	No significant differences were found between groups for student delays, although a trend favoring in-class condition was found
Palisano (1989)	Comparison of PT and OT in groups via direct service and consultation; teacher satisfaction	Progress of 34 elementary students with learning disabilities compared on three motor and visual-motor tests	Each group made greater change on one measure; both groups made comparable progress on third measure
Dunn (1990)	Comparison of direct service and consultation; teacher and therapist attitudes surveyed	14 preschoolers were randomly assigned to either group; IEP goal attainment used to measure outcomes	Children in both groups achieved a similar percentage of IEP goals; teachers in consultation group reported larger OT contributions and more positive attitudes

Developing a Consultation Plan

Once you have collected information about a student's abilities and functional problems, the learning environment, and available human resources, you should develop a plan of action. This plan will guide your consultation, just as you would develop a treatment plan for direct intervention. We have designed a reproducible School Consultation Plan to guide your thinking and record your observations as you gather data to plan intervention (see figure 8.1, pages 123-124). Use the blank reproducible School Consultation Plan provided on pages 148-149 of the appendix as a mental guide or complete it in writing; however, always develop your plan with other team members' input. Each section of the form is described below.

1. ***When and where the consulting therapist will observe/assess/work with student***

   Specify where and when you will observe or work with a particular student. The School Consultation Plan is applicable even if you are working with a student individually in the classroom or other school area. (Remember that direct service should always be paired with consultation with other team members.)

2. ***When and where the consulting therapist will meet with team members***

   After seeing a student, you will need to find time to discuss your observations and suggestions with team members. Refer to the suggested strategies for scheduling discussion time described previously in this chapter (pages 108 to 109).

3. ***Student's strengths***

   The important data you collected during stage two of the consulting process (issue definition) included looking at the abilities and strengths of the student. We have provided a section on the form to summarize this information as a reminder that your recommendations should build on whatever abilities the student possesses. This information can help other team members view the student positively; you will gain a new perspective of the student also.

4. ***Student's functional problems***

   Functional is the key word in the development of your consultation plan. Keep in mind that your ultimate goal is to help students improve their school performance. Avoid summarizing problems in medical terms. Look at how your traditional therapy concerns affect educational performance (chapter 2). Translate your clinical knowledge into language that is more useful in a school-based setting. For example, Shirley is a 5-year-old student with mental retardation. Instead of noting her clinical deficits as "Delayed grasp, release, and in-hand manipulation skills due to problems with intrinsic hand muscles," summarize Shirley's functional problems this way, "Can't fasten buttons, hold a pencil, or cut with scissors." Her difficulty with intrinsic hand muscles is the cause of her functional problems, which you must consider when making recommendations to improve her performance.

5. ***Student's educational outcomes***

   Once you have identified the student's functional problems in the school setting, translate them into desired educational outcomes. Include outcomes that you and other team members have identified. The temptation at this point may be to identify that "Shirley needs physical or occupational therapy twice a week." However, physical and occupational therapy are not educational outcomes; they are important services that can help students enhance their performance in school lessons and activities.

6. ***Recommendations***

   Next you should list strategies to help the student achieve desired outcomes. Ask yourself, "How can I help Shirley complete her art and other class projects?" You may tentatively decide that Shirley should use a small pair of scissors and heavyweight construction paper when she cuts so the paper will not flop over her hand. You recommend consultation with the assistant teacher to show how to set up the task as well as position Shirley to use her hands to best advantage.

7. ***Follow-up plan***

   The final section of the form is for specifying how you will provide follow-up support; in particular, how often and at what time of day. For Shirley, you recommend consultation with the classroom assistant once per month.

At the conclusion of stage 2 (issue definition) of the consulting process, you should meet with other team members to develop or review an IEP for your student. You can use the School Consultation Plan at this meeting to share your observations and recommendations with your team and develop a final consultation plan. Legally, your proposed recommendations are just that, proposed, until the team has had a chance to jointly decide on a plan for the student. Unfortunately, in some school systems the IEP meeting has become a pro forma approval of disciplinary goals and objectives before a thorough description of the student's educational outcomes are discussed. Developing isolated PT and OT goals and objectives for the IEP and stapling them together for parents' approval not only discourages collaborative consultation but defeats the intent and requirements of the Individuals with Disabilities Education Act. In a Notice of Interpretation of IEP Requirements, the U. S. Department of Education described the purpose of an IEP:

> There are two main parts of the IEP requirements, as described in the Act and regulations: (1) The IEP meeting(s), where parents and school personnel jointly make decisions about an educational program for a child with a disability, and (2) the IEP document itself, that is, a written record of the decisions reached at the meeting.
>
> Appendix C to 34 C.F.R. Part 300, Response to Question No. 55

The Notice of Interpretation specifically states that:

> It is not permissible for an agency to present a completed IEP to parents for their approval before there has been a full discussion with the parents of (1) the child's need for special education and related services, and (2) what services the agency will provide to the child.
>
> Appendix to Part 330, Question No. 55

You can still meet the intent of the law and best practice for collaborative consultation by preparing your detailed notes on the School Consultation Plan regarding a student's strengths, functional problems, and suggested educational outcomes and convey this information during an IEP development meeting with your team.

Conclusion

This chapter discussed how to turn administrative and personal barriers to consultation into opportunities to enlist family and educator support and plan for system-wide change. One final word, from a wise statesman, warns about taking on more than you can really accomplish by yourself:

> To get the bad customs of a country changed and new ones, though better, introduced, it is necessary first to remove the prejudices of the people, enlighten their ignorance, and convince them that their interests will be promoted by the proposed changes; and this is not the work of a day.
>
> Benjamin Franklin, quoted in Rogers 1983

Changing behavior, expectations, and attitudes in order to expand your delivery of physical and occupational therapy is not the work of one day. Plan ahead, enlist support, and give yourself ample time to put your vision into action.

Selected Readings

Bennis, W., K. Benne, R. Chin, and K. Corey, Eds. 1976. *The planning of change.* New York: Holt, Rinehart and Winston.

Rogers, E. 1983. *Diffusion of innovation,* 3d ed. New York: The Free Press.

These classic textbooks on change discuss crucial factors to consider before implementing new consultative therapy services in the schools; for example, initiating new programs in human systems, facilitating a shared commitment to change, and disseminating information about new programs and ideas to win support. Although not directed specifically at change in the school system, the authors provide much food for thought about starting new programs and changing ideas.

Eitington, J. 1989. *The winning trainer,* 2d ed. Houston: Gulf.

This book is a comprehensive collection of training and facilitation strategies and activities that is very useful for school-based therapists who are planning inservices and other presentations.

Johnson, J., M. Pugach, and D. Hammittee. 1988. Barriers to effective special education consultation. *Remedial and Special Education* 9(6):41-47.

This article provides a succinct summary of the barriers to effective consultation facing educators. These barriers should also be considered by consulting therapists.

Figure 8.1

School Consultation Plan

Student's name: Shirley Age: 5 years Date: December 12

Collaborators: Jill Martin Role: Teacher

Fran Collingsworth Role: OT

Janice Barton Role: Mother

1. When and where the consulting therapist will observe/assess/work with the student:

Dates:	Where (classroom, PE, lunch, recess, bathroom, other)?
December 10	Classroom during art project (10 a.m.) Center time (10:20 a.m.)

2. When the consulting therapist will meet with team members for planning:

Dates:	Who? At what time?
December 8	Teacher and mother at 3:30 p.m. in classroom

3. Student's strengths (observed by educational team and consulting therapist):

- Loves playground equipment—climbs and swings well.
- Very social—has many friends.
- Is interested in classroom pets.
- Has good auditory memory.

4. Student's functional problems (observed by educational team and consulting therapist):

- Can't fasten buttons, hold a pencil, or cut with scissors.
- Doesn't like art or coloring.
- Is confused by simple worksheets.
- Switches hands when using paint brush/crayons.

5. Student's desired educational outcomes (describe desired performance/behavior):

- Recognize and copy shapes (square, triangle) and letters.
- Cut construction paper for art projects.
- Use a consistent hand to color and paint.

6. Recommendations for intervention:

What to try:	Who will do it?	When?
• Gather data about preferred hand.	Assistant teacher with OT input	December 15
• Use heavyweight construction paper and small scissors when cutting.	Assistant teacher/mother	Ongoing activity
• Copy and color on vertical surfaces (blackboard, easel).	Assistant teacher/mother	Ongoing activity

7. Follow-up plan

How will consulting therapist follow up?	When?
• Develop chart for recording data about hand use.	By December 15
• Complete visual-motor assessment.	By December 15
• Observe in classroom/meet with teacher and assistant on monthly basis.	Every 3rd Monday (10 a.m.)

In this chapter we:

- identify potential conflicts that may arise during the various phases of consultation
- discuss and model strategies to address these conflicts
- recommend ways to practice conflict resolution skills

Chapter 9

Conflict Resolution

> *It takes two to tangle, but it takes only one to begin to untangle a knotty situation. It is within your power to transform even your most difficult relationships. Your greatest power is the power to change the game—from face-to-face confrontation to side-by-side joint problem solving.*
>
> Ury 1993

Consultation can be a stimulating and rewarding experience as you work with team members to enhance a student's performance in school. Sharing an "Ah-ha!" experience with a teacher or family member as your efforts come together for a student is one of the rewards of consulting. However, there are challenges that you will face on this path to success. Interactions among you and other team members make consulting complex as well as rewarding. We have identified the major challenges that may occur during each of the four stages of the consulting process. In the section entitled Lessons Learned at the conclusion of each section, we identify consulting challenges and suggest resolutions.

Consulting with another team member often means that you will ask for changes in the team member's behavior. Such a request can be difficult, no matter how much change is desired by all parties. Knowing that interpersonal difficulties frequently occur can assist you in dealing with them. The important point to keep in mind is that these confrontations are natural and predictable.

Resolving conflicts about consulting services and student programs is actually a form of negotiation. All involved parties discuss their concerns and suggestions and negotiate to come to a mutually satisfactory resolution. This negotiation is essential for two main reasons:

- The therapist wants to implement the program that is the most appropriate for the student.
- The program is going to be carried out by another person who must be convinced that the recommended approach is best.

Negotiation is a complex skill but one that therapists can acquire or refine through study and practice. Fisher and Ury (1983, 36) provide a useful metaphor for thinking about negotiation.

> It is easy sometimes to forget that a negotiation is not a debate. Nor is it a trial. You are not trying to persuade some third party. The person you are trying to persuade is seated at the table with you. If a negotiation is to be compared with a legal proceeding, the situation resembles that of two judges trying to reach agreement on how to decide a case. Try putting yourself in that role, treating your opposite number as a fellow judge with whom you are attempting to work out a joint opinion. In this context it is clearly unpersuasive to blame the other party for the problem, to engage in name-calling, or to raise your voice. On the contrary, it will help to recognize explicitly that they see the situation differently and to try to go forward as people with a joint problem.

Conflict management and negotiation is not a malady that must be endured. Dealing with conflicts successfully can be beneficial to the team and to the individuals. Some of the positive outcomes of successful conflict resolution that have been cited in the literature include:

- improved relationships among the team members
- enhanced feelings of self-confidence, competence, self-worth, and power (Dettmer, Thurston, and Dyck 1993)
- increased motivation among the team members involved in the conflict
- increased perspective-taking
- higher levels of cognitive reasoning
- more creativity
- increased quality in problem solving
- higher levels of satisfaction among the team members who make decisions and follow through with them (Idol, Nevin, and Paolucci-Whitcomb 1994)

Stage 1: Entry—Typical Interpersonal Conflicts

Effective consultation is easier if good relationships are developed in the very beginning of the consultation process. Establishing positive relationships can be difficult, especially for a therapist who is inexperienced in consulting or an experienced therapist who is new to a school or works in many different schools each week. The start of a new school year is always somewhat hectic. You may decide that other tasks have priority over "chatting" with team members or potential team members. This misperception may lead to future problems.

A consulting therapist's first priority is to establish positive relationships with faculty, staff, families, and administrators. As internationally renowned negotiators Fisher and Ury (1983) stated, "The best time for handling people problems is before they become people problems. This means building a personal and organizational relationship with the other side that can cushion the people on each side against the knocks of negotiation" (p. 38). Each new consulting situation and relationship will demand different actions on your part, but all should start with the explicit goal of establishing positive relationships. Plan time during each day to get to know a new team member better, strengthen a blossoming relationship, or reinforce an established friendship. Ask yourself at the end of each school day, "What did I do today to improve my relationship with a colleague or a family member?" Record your accomplishments just as you would document therapy sessions and number of students served.

Sometimes, despite your best efforts, you may encounter problems establishing a positive relationship. Your team member may have had negative experiences with a prior consultant or may have other reasons to be hesitant, or even hostile, to you as the new consulting therapist. The following suggestions are helpful for dealing with these initial conflict situations.

Think before You Speak

One of the most challenging situations you will experience during the Entry stage is an uncooperative team member who lacks interest in your consultation. The team member may not even want to spend time getting to know you or find out what you have to offer. Feeling miffed at this rejection, you may be tempted to say, "You have to do what I say because it's on the IEP!" Keep in mind that there are other alternatives to relying on authority. Ury (1993, 160) discusses this human reaction and reminds consultants of their goal.

> Your goal is not to win over them, but to win them over. To accomplish this goal, you need to resist normal human temptations and do the opposite of what you naturally feel like doing. You need to suspend your reaction when you feel like striking back, to ask questions when you feel like telling your opponents the answers, to bridge your differences when you feel like pushing for your way, and to educate when you feel like escalating.

Model Openness

Regardless of the initial interactions, always prepare yourself for future differences of opinion and take action early on to set the stage for effective management of conflict. You want to be viewed as a professional who seeks constructive criticism, is open to suggestions, and strives to improve knowledge and skills. If you model these attitudes early on, when other team members disagree with a recommendation or how a program is working out, they will feel comfortable bringing this up to you without feeling that they are hurting your pride or reputation.

Be Respectful

Respect all team members. If you must collaborate with a teacher who is less than enthusiastic about consulting with you, be especially careful to show respect and to minimize intrusion. We have discussed some rules of etiquette in chapter 4 that will be especially useful for establishing a positive relationship under difficult circumstances. Try to understand the teacher's viewpoint and predict reactions to help you optimize your interactions. For example, if you must work with a student outside of the classroom, ask when the student's absence would be least upsetting to the class schedule. Try to respect the teacher's wishes about meeting times and when and where you observe the student. Any gesture on your part to meet the teacher more than halfway will indicate that you are there to provide assistance and support.

Pay Sincere Compliments

Compliments go a long way in establishing rapport but work only if they are sincere. The more specific the compliment, the stronger its impact. Perhaps you observed a particularly positive interaction between a teacher and student when you were with another class on the playground. You might comment to the teacher, "The way you organized the Olympic games so that you could involve Jamie was very impressive. She was obviously having a great time while gaining strength and confidence." Even under the most difficult circumstances, if you look hard enough, there is always something positive to draw attention to; for instance, the way the environment is arranged reflects the values or aesthetics of the team member. For instance, "I always enjoy coming into your class and seeing the students' artwork so creatively displayed on the bulletin boards." This might be the very icebreaker that is needed in this particular relationship. Once some of the hostility decreases, you may be pleasantly surprised to discover other positive aspects that you previously overlooked.

Transform Strained Relationships

The methods you will use to bridge your differences with a team member will vary depending on your personality and style as well as those of the team member. You might consider the following strategies:

- Engage the team member in conversation about unrelated topics such as an upcoming school event or vacation.
- Discreetly seek insights about the team member from others.
- Ask the team member for advice about something unrelated to your conflict.
- Try to understand the underlying rationale for the strained interaction from all perspectives.

Once you start thinking creatively, you can come up with ways to improve this relationship. Sometimes you can do this indirectly. You might drop by before school starts and ask if you can help set up one of the study areas. You might research a topic that interests the teacher and offer some of the materials you have found. Perhaps you can bring treats on Halloween. Talking with your supervisor or with other team members discreetly may give you insights into ways to improve your relationship with this person. You might ask the teacher for suggestions or advice about an unrelated issue. If you are new to a community, you might ask the teacher for some kind of assistance; for instance, "Would you know where I can get farm fresh vegetables?" Sometimes you need to probe to discover the underlying causes for the strained relationship. Perhaps the team member has had negative experiences with other consultants that influence interactions with you.

What is most important is to establish a positive relationship, even if it seems difficult. "An important strategy for dealing with resistance and defensiveness is to handle your own defensiveness, stop pushing so that the other person will not be able to push back, delay reactions, keep quiet, and listen. This takes practice, patience, tolerance, and commitment" (Dettmer, Thurston, and Dyck 1993, 174).

Lessons Learned

You drop by Georgia's room before class starts to talk about Soon Hee and ask when it would be convenient for you to observe him. Georgia tells you that she wants you there at 10:00 a.m. You utter a mental "uh-oh" because you have a standing appointment with a teacher in another school at that time. When you tell Georgia of this conflict, she retorts, "Why do you therapists even bother to ask what I want when you're just going to do what you want anyway?" Knowing how overburdened your schedule is, you want to say that she should be happy you even bothered to ask. However, you take a moment to think about why this seemingly innocent conversation has turned into a conflict. Instead of reacting, you find out why Georgia wants you to observe the student at 10 a.m. "If I understand correctly, you want me to observe Soon Hee's gross motor skills. I'd like to come at 10, when you are on the playground, but I have a conflict. When is Soon Hee in PE? That's perfect. Do you think I could observe him then and get back to you later with my observations?"

The therapist in this situation showed respect by asking about the teacher's preferences. During a difficult encounter she thought before she spoke and she transformed a strained relationship by seeking further information about the teacher's need. She then offered an alternative that would meet both their needs.

Roy has been consulting for less than two years and is starting a new consultative relationship with Sandy, who has been teaching for almost 20 years. Roy notices that Sandy goes out of her way to be supportive and never makes negative comments. Roy asks Sandy to meet with him after school. "Sandy, I have a favor to ask you. I'm not in this building very often since Emil is my only student here. Both of us have to make an effort to share progress and problems that we encounter as Emil is integrated into your shop class. I know that you have been the head vocational education teacher for a long time and I admit I don't know the rules and procedures of a vocational education class. I'm a little concerned that I might break some class rules or interfere with your routines. I sure hope you'll warn me or let me know if I do.

In this scenario, the therapist made sure to establish a relationship with frank and open communication. This is the best way to prepare for dealing with conflicts that might emerge later in the relationship. The therapist also acknowledged the teacher's long service and the leadership role she has earned—a good foundation for the development of a positive relationship.

Practicing Negotiation Skills

Identify a person, such as a teacher, relative, or friend, with whom you have a strained relationship. Observe this person unobtrusively and look for positive behaviors or attributes. Jot down compliments you could legitimately pay this person and, if you feel comfortable doing so, share them. Pay close attention to your feelings and the reactions of the person you are complimenting.

Stage 2: Identifying the Issue—Typical Interpersonal Conflicts

Your first encounter with formal negotiations will probably occur when planning new services or a new approach for a student. Each team member at the planning table may have strong opinions and commitments to the student. Each of you also has different goals, methods, and values. One or more members of the team may disagree with your opinions and perhaps with each other's ideas as well. You could view this conflict as an impediment to effective consultation or as an opportunity to consider new options for helping the student. "Opposite types may or may not attract, but they definitely need to be present for greatest team productivity. Such differences can be useful, but managing them elegantly is a tremendous challenge for a consultant or a consulting teacher" (Dettmer, Thurston, and Dyck 1993, 113).

How do you succeed despite this challenge? You can usually avoid an impasse in a meeting by following the guidelines for stage 2, Issue Definition, discussed in chapter 7. Infrequently, the team will be in total disagreement and you might need to lead the team through a negotiation process. Your first task is to defuse any contention and then get the team moving to the task of addressing the needs of the student. Your goal is to assist your fellow team members to focus on the student, not on their disagreements.

The following scenarios model some of the skills that are useful for negotiating a mutually acceptable conclusion. The skills that are modeled include:

- identifying communication mistakes as soon as possible
- establishing and maintaining effective nonverbal communication
- expressing genuine respect and admiration for others
- recognizing the other's contributions
- refocusing on student needs and outcomes
- understanding the rationale for other team members' requests
- paraphrasing or restating discussion as needed to assure mutual understanding
- steering the conversation back on track

Lessons Learned

LaKeisha was initially evaluated at a local hospital where the staff were unfamiliar with educationally relevant therapy. The hospital-based therapist, Lorna, attends LaKeisha's IEP meeting and recommends therapy four times a week. Marguerite, the school therapist, believes there is no rationale for this level of service in the school setting. She explains the educational process to Lorna, who dismisses Marguerite's experience by commenting, "I've worked in a hospital for 17 years and you've worked in the schools for only three years." Holding back a retort, Marguerite takes a deep breath and asks to review Lorna's evaluations and recommendations. This action not only gives Marguerite more information but allows her to calm down and deal with her feelings.

Marguerite did not react negatively to the provocation. Instead, she found a way to buy time by reviewing Lorna's written reports during which she composed herself before proceeding with the discussion.

Marguerite and two educators along with the school principal and LaKeisha's mother, Mrs. Brown, are developing goals and objectives for LaKeisha's IEP. Marguerite has just finished describing LaKeisha's motor planning difficulties in layman's terms and asks LaKeisha's mother if she has any suggestions for what she wants LaKeisha to accomplish. Mrs. Brown states emphatically that she wants LaKeisha to be able to tie her own shoes as soon as possible. Marguerite doubts if LaKeisha will be able to tie her shoes this year and suggests another objective. LaKeisha's mother becomes very upset. "I knew I shouldn't have bothered coming to this meeting. You're just like the people at LaKeisha's former school. You pretend to listen and then just write me off."

Marguerite leans across the table, looks at LaKeisha's mother, and says, "I am very sorry, Mrs. Brown. I shouldn't have denied your request before we had a chance to talk about it. We've all been impressed by your involvement in LaKeisha's education and your concern for her success in school. We all want to see her progress. As her mother, you know many things about LaKeisha that we don't." Mrs. Brown sits back in her chair. "Well, nothing is more important to me than my child's well-being." Marguerite acknowledges her comment by saying, "I understand that having LaKeisha tie her own shoes is important to you. Can you help me understand why you want her to do this now?" Mrs. Brown replies, "I remember when each of my children first tied their own shoes. To me, it was a sign they were growing up and on the road to independence." Marguerite listens and acknowledges Mrs. Brown's feelings by saying, "So tying her own shoes is a sign of independence for LaKeisha." Mrs. Brown nods and Marguerite exclaims energetically, "Well, let's see how we can promote LaKeisha's independence," and everyone joins in the task.

In this case, Marguerite quickly recognized her mistake and acknowledged it. She re-established communication with Mrs. Brown by leaning toward her and establishing eye contact. She expressed her genuine respect for Mrs. Brown's participation in LaKeisha's education and recognized her contribution to the planning process. Marguerite tried to understand the rationale behind Mrs. Brown's request and restated her concern for two reasons: to make sure she accurately understood the request and to give it legitimacy. Finally, Marguerite moved the focus back to LaKeisha and encouraged the team to return to their planning activity with renewed vigor and enthusiasm.

Practicing Negotiation Skills

Read one or more of the texts from the selected readings at the end of this chapter for further information about negotiating skills. Make a list of the techniques you think are particularly useful and then write each one on an index card. Think of a difficult situation in which you were unhappy with the outcome. Ask a friend to reenact the situation with you, playing the role of the person whom you perceived to be the adversary. As you begin the role play, select an index card at random and for two minutes practice the negotiation skill listed. Do not let your friend see the card. Repeat this procedure several times throughout your role play. When you have finished, talk with your friend about how the various negotiating techniques affected your interaction.

Stage 3: Implementing Recommendations—Typical Interpersonal Conflicts

At some point in your consulting experience, you will disagree with how another team member carries out the intervention that the team has agreed upon. You may think it is not being done right or often enough, or maybe not at all. Anticipate such conflicts between what you expected and what actually happens, as they are inevitable. "It is unrealistic to expect all classroom teachers to adopt instructional modifications comfortably and willingly . . . It is human nature to be uncomfortable when another person disagrees. It is also human nature to get upset when someone resists efforts to make changes, implement plans, or modify systems to be more responsive to students' special needs" (Dettmer, Thurston, and Dyck 1993).

Keep in mind that it is your recommendations, not you personally, that are the central focus of the conflict. Most likely, the teacher misunderstood your suggestions, the student's situation changed, or your recommendations need modification. We have used three stress-reducers successfully in these types of situations:

- Never jump to conclusions.
- Assume the best, until that rare situation when you find otherwise; that is, assume that the team member really wants what is best for the student.
- Identify and deal with your feelings before you approach a team member with whom you disagree unless you have a strong and established relationship. This might be a good time to let off steam with a friend or supervisor first.

Restoring your perspective will prepare you to handle this challenging situation. Gather more information before you take any action. Judiciously solicit feedback from your team members about how your suggestions are working out by asking questions such as:

- How well do you think this process is working?
- What progress have you seen in the student as a result of the consulting interventions?
- What features of this program do you think are the most beneficial? Which are the least helpful or most demanding?
- What changes would you suggest?

These nonadversarial, information-seeking questions can lead you to understand your team members' viewpoints about how your recommendations are working. If a team member shares your dissatisfaction, your job will be much easier because you both desire change. You can build upon this motivation for change. "Why do you think John hasn't made the progress we anticipated?" If you have established a positive relationship, the teacher can share discontent without fearing that your feelings will be hurt.

If your team members are satisfied with how they implement your suggestions but you are not, your situation is different. You will need to share your expectations and observations and reach an agreement with them about modifying the intervention. Identify the discrepancy between your expectations and their actual implementation. Given new information, team members may accept your viewpoint and immediately modify the student's program.

You must also be open to the possibility that your intervention is too complex, developmentally inappropriate, or too hard to implement. Resistance to your program may indicate that there are real issues to attend to and you may be the one who must make some changes to the recommendations. Team members may resist implementing your recommendations for several reasons. They may:

- have too little or inaccurate information about the intervention
- disagree about assessment or intervention methods and activities
- maintain a difference of opinion regarding goals and desired outcomes

(Dettmer, Thurston, and Dyck 1993)

Probe carefully to determine why the program is not being implemented as designed. Once you identify the issue, you can determine the best course of action. If the problem is too little or inaccurate information, you can easily provide it. If the team member disagrees with your intervention or desired outcome, you need to focus on what changes will improve student performance. An effective method to resolve this type of conflict is to understand the team member's perceptions. "What do you think will motivate Carlos to use his prosthesis?" Reaffirm that you are interested in helping the teacher and the student. "We all want Carlos to move around the classroom easily. Let's put our heads together and figure out what we can do to accomplish this." The goal is a win/win compromise, with all team members feeling good about the interaction. Successful negotiation requires:

- dealing effectively with your own emotions
- helping to defuse the other party's negative reactions
- confirming a commitment to solve the problem without damaging the relationship
- engaging in joint problem solving and coming to agreement about the best possible option

(Ury 1993)

Learning to negotiate may be difficult but can also be extremely rewarding. How can you develop and refine your negotiation skills? As a start, read the resources in the suggested readings list at the end of this chapter. You may also want to check into courses at your local university or college for additional training in this area.

Sometimes a peer support system is an ideal way to review the effectiveness of particularly challenging situations and to learn from others' experiences. Self-reflection is also an important way to monitor your interaction techniques and identify the strengths and skills you desire to acquire.

Lessons Learned

All parties at the IEP meeting have agreed that Nigel needs to increase his time in the prone stander. Karl, the school therapist, proposes that Alison, the classroom assistant, learn to position Nigel with his training and supervision. Karl returns for his scheduled follow-up two weeks after providing the training. Alison reports that they have not had time to use the stander because they were so busy with the holidays and other classroom events. Karl asks Alison why positioning Nigel has been so difficult and how she has tried to overcome the problem. Listening carefully, he realizes that Alison thinks Nigel is uncomfortable in the prone stander and she does not want to place him in it for longer periods.

First, Karl acknowledges Alison's concerns and then asks her for suggestions. She proposes that he take Nigel to the therapy room for the extra time. Karl knows this option will not work for several reasons. He cannot see Nigel every day, Nigel would miss too much class time, and Alison would never learn to use the prone stander. He suggests, instead, "What if we watch a videotape about prone standers together?" Karl also knows some teachers and students who are very satisfied with the same equipment. He arranges for them to talk with Alison about their experiences. Afterward, she still hesitates to use the stander. Karl explains how Nigel will benefit from daily use of the prone stander and Alison agrees these outcomes are important. You concur, "Okay, we're in agreement about what Nigel needs. Let's review our options for meeting them." At the conclusion of the discussion, Karl summarizes their agreement. "Let's confirm what we're going to try. I will come in and work with you to position Nigel and will stay until he's ready to sit back in his wheelchair. You'll try to position him in the prone stander every day for the first week. I'll be back next Tuesday. If you have any concerns before then, you'll call me. Is this an accurate summary of our plan?"

Karl dealt with this conflict by asking problem-solving questions, such as, "Why?" "Why not?" and "What if?" He also asked for team members' suggestions. Remember to work as a team to solve any dilemma; that is, move from a you-versus-me attitude to a let's-solve-this-together plan (Ury 1993). In this scenario, Karl negotiated by focusing on their shared agreement about Nigel's needs and by using phrases such as "our plan" and "we agree."

Practicing Negotiation Skills

Rent a video, preferably one you have already seen, or watch a television show with a friend who does not mind talking during the show. Notice conflict between the characters and identify how they attempt to resolve it. Identify both useful and not-so-useful attempts. Decide if the conflict was resolved successfully. How did all parties feel at the conclusion of the negotiation? Was the conflict solved? Figure 9.1 summarizes the strategies discussed in this chapter to guide your analysis.

Figure 9.1
Strategies for Successful Negotiation

Stage 1, Entry, focused on developing a positive relationship:

- Think before you speak when in a potentially eruptive discussion.
- Model openness.
- Be respectful.
- Transform strained relationships by finding neutral interests.

Stage 2, Issue Definition, highlighted how to use these effective communication and negotiation skills:

- Identify communication mistakes early.
- Establish and maintain nonverbal communication.
- Express genuine respect and admiration.
- Recognize others' contributions.
- Refocus on student abilities, needs, and desired outcomes.
- Understand the rationale for team members' requests and concerns.
- Restate discussion to ensure mutual understanding.

Stage 3, Implementing Recommendations, emphasized the following problem-solving strategies:

- Identify your feelings before confronting team members.
- Defuse negative reactions by acknowledging them in yourself and others.
- Be willing to modify your intervention when it does not appear successful.
- Reaffirm that you are all members of a team with more agreements than disagreements.
- Reestablish common ground regarding student outcomes and intervention strategies.
- Ask problem-solving questions such as, "what if?" "why?" and "what else?"

Stage 4: Concluding—Typical Interpersonal Conflicts

At this stage, there are two reasons for pausing and reflecting on your consultation. The first involves reaching closure on a specific consulting objective and the second involves concluding the consultative relationship. *Closure* occurs when the team decides that a student's educational outcome has been accomplished and it may help you identify other educational outcomes to work on together. You should take the lead in making the recommendation for closure, discussing the completed outcomes with the team and proposing new educational outcomes. At this point, you would cycle back to Stage 2, Issue Definition.

Conclusion occurs when you complete a program or finish the consulting relationship for some other reason, such as the end of the school year. The most important responsibility during this stage is to ensure the team members are in agreement that all of the objectives have been addressed and that the consultation will end.

In most situations, team members will agree that your consultation was successful and that the student's needs have been met. Some consulting relationships will be more difficult to conclude than others, especially if you believe the time has come to conclude the consultation and others disagree. Disagreement might stem from the concern that the student has not made sufficient progress, or team members may want your continued support.

In addition, some family members may resist ending consultation. They may think that the therapist is giving up or that if the consultation continued, their child could make still more progress. The best way to prevent problems during the concluding stage is to keep all parties informed on a regular basis from the very beginning about progress and expectations. Preparing family and other team members for the conclusion of consultation is one of your primary responsibilities through all stages of the consultation relationship.

If, after appropriate preparation, a team member still expresses a concern, some negotiation may be necessary. Some strategies for alleviating anxieties are:

- requesting a neutral third-party opinion
- assuring continued availability
- acknowledging and addressing unmet needs
- offering encouragement that team members are capable of handling the situation on their own

Perhaps you can request that another school therapist observe and evaluate the student. If this second therapist corroborates your recommendation, it might allay the anxieties of the family or other team member. Another option you might choose is to assure the team that you are still available if concerns arise and can return in a specified time period to observe the student.

Sometimes this transition brings up unstated concerns of your team members. Avoid allowing team members to become overly dependent on you so you can minimize the loss incurred when you end the consulting relationship. However, no matter what you do, some team members will miss the camaraderie of shared interactions and the stimulus of professional input. You can assist the team by introducing colleagues or family members who have been dealing with similar circumstances or link a newcomer who wants to learn a specific skill with the teacher who has refined that skill during the year. To ease transition anxieties, you might point out how well things are going and compliment the team on their accomplishments.

When you conclude a consulting relationship with a student, you should expect and prepare for some negative as well as positive feelings. Students may have contradictory feelings, perhaps feeling proud to have "graduated" from therapy but sorry to be losing a supportive adult. Be prepared to deal with "acting out" or unpredictable behavior. You can minimize problems by keeping students informed and letting students participate in the plan for ending consultation. This planning will vary depending on the skills of students. You might set up a pictorial calendar for nonreaders. Others might like the idea of a diary to record progress and anticipated dates for concluding your consultation. Some students may just need to talk about the upcoming transition. Your responsibility is to inquire about and assist students with acknowledging and dealing with any feelings about the conclusion of your relationships.

You may also be sorry to leave the relationship and need to recognize your own feelings while keeping the needs of the student and your team members as your first priority. Be careful that your feelings do not influence your professional judgment. For example, do not prolong consultation beyond what you think is appropriate because you do not want to leave the team or because you are afraid of another team member's reaction. Perhaps the most challenging situation during this final stage is to decide when to actually end the consultation. Your decision should be determined by whether or not the educational outcome the team decided upon has been achieved. The student may still have poor balance or low muscle tone; however, the question is whether or not the student's educational performance has improved. Standards for medical treatment are not the same as for educational therapy. If you believe that everything has been done to meet the student's educational outcomes, you need to actively begin concluding the consultation. An effective team will have specified these outcomes during the planning phase.

No matter what the circumstances, try to conclude your relationship with some positive ritual (Gallesich 1982). Even under the most difficult of leave-takings, you might write a note of appreciation to each team member, including the student, emphasizing at least one positive experience. Most experiences will be very positive and you might take the initiative to hold a party to celebrate the student's progress and the positive relationships you all have experienced.

Lessons Learned

Sheryl has been providing therapy to Donita for two years, pairing direct service with consultation in the classroom. Sheryl feels like she is part of the classroom staff, but she realizes she must think about what to recommend for next year. Donita has met her goals and further therapy is unlikely to result in educationally relevant progress. However, Sheryl is concerned that she might be missing possible objectives or there might be an intervention she has not tried. She asks a colleague to review her program and observe Donita. Afterward, her colleague confirms that therapy would probably not result in further gains at this time. While talking, Sheryl realizes how much she has enjoyed her work with Donita and her teachers and family. Her colleague concurs, "I've been in relationships like this, too, where everything is going so well you don't want to change anything. You've done a fine job of making everyone feel comfortable and involved."

Sheryl realizes that it is time to end her consultative services. Her colleague shares how she concludes her own consultations by throwing a party so that everyone, including the student and her family, can celebrate the student's graduation from therapy. Sheryl likes this idea and plans to make funny party favors for each member of the team. She is especially interested in Donita's reaction to the poster she has made of fun and challenging situations that occurred during therapy.

In this scenario, Sheryl employed good listening skills, used a neutral party for an independent opinion, sought out unmet feelings, offered compliments for achievements, and celebrated successes.

Practicing Negotiation Skills

1. Review chapter 2 to reassess the differences between the educational model and the medical model. Review your current consultation roster and determine if any students have accomplished their educational outcomes. If appropriate, begin the process of concluding therapy for these students.

2. Talk with other therapists, teachers, and family members about their experiences with concluding consultation. Ask them to comment on the "best of times" and the "worst of times." Decide which activities and traditions match your personality and the characteristics of your team and try them out.

Conclusion

Providing services as a consulting therapist can be a rewarding experience as team members share the pleasures of success and work out conflicts. However, the same relationships that provide these pleasures also present consulting's greatest challenges. You must work with and through team members to carry out your recommendations. Collaborative consultation often leads to a better plan and program for the student and to improved functioning of the team, but there are likely to be difficult moments when team members disagree with one another. We have described conflict resolution as a negotiation process, identified some of the common conflicts that are likely to emerge during each stage of consultation, and suggested strategies that might be useful for addressing these challenges. Learning to negotiate is difficult work, but the results of successfully coming to a mutually supportive resolution can be most satisfying.

Selected Readings

Dettmer, P., L. Thurston, and N. Dyck. 1993. *Consultation, collaboration and teamwork for students with special needs*. Boston: Allyn and Bacon.

Chapter 6 of this book focuses on communication skills and describes many excellent strategies for managing resistance, anger, and conflict among team members in an education setting. Chapter 11 is devoted to consulting and collaborating in partnerships with parents and offers tips for establishing good relationships in order to deter future conflict.

Fisher, R., and W. Ury. 1983. *Getting to yes*. New York: Penguin Books.

This short book is a must-read for all people who interact with others and offers easily understood strategies for coming to mutually satisfying resolutions. The authors' information is useful regardless of the type of conflict or setting in which they occur. The book's main premise is that to be successful, all parties of the conflict should be able to win. The basic steps are to separate the people from the problem, focus on interests not positions, invent options for mutual gain, and insist on using objective criteria.

Ury, W. 1993. *Getting past no: Negotiating your way from confrontation to cooperation.* New York: Bantam Books.

This book, by one of the authors of *Getting to yes,* presents useful information about how to deal with roadblocks and other barriers during negotiation. Some of the topics include staying in control when in a confrontational situation, defusing your own and others' hostility and anger, finding out what the other side really wants, and reaching agreements that satisfy both sides' needs. Every consulting therapist can benefit from reading this interesting book.

Appendix
Reproducible Forms

Observing Student Performance in School*

Student: ______________________ Age: __________ Date: ______________

Observed by: ____

Activity observed: ____

The following questions provide a framework for observing a student in school. The focus of the questions is on behavior and skills that are viewed by educators as essential for successful performance in school.

Performance Parameters	Comments
A. Purpose of Task	
1. Academic or nonacademic subject or area? 2. Objective of lesson/activity? 3. Relationship to student's IEP goals/objectives?	
B. Nature of Activity	
1. Individual, paired, or group? 2. Therapeutic domains (motor, perceptual, neuromuscular, sensory processing, adaptive behavior)? 3. Sensory input inherent in task?	
C. Accuracy of Performance	
1. Which parts of task can student do? 2. Which parts are difficult? 3. Does student compensate? How?	
D. Attention to Activity	
1. Length of attention to task? 2. Distracted? By what stimuli or event? 3. Can refocus attention if interrupted?	
E. Handling Transitions	
1. From one activity to another? 2. Within areas of the classroom/school? 3. Has previous activity affected performance?	

Materials created by Barbara Hanft and Patricia Place.

Performance Parameters	Comments
F. Problem Solving	
1. Understands and follows directions? 2. Has plan of what to do? 3. Makes changes if difficulty arises?	
G. Organization	
1. Desk, cubby, backpack (3-D space)? 2. Papers and workbooks (2-D space)? 3. Knows schedule and class routines?	
H. Posture/Motor	
1. Comfortable, upright posture for seat work? 2. Functional self-help and playground skills? 3. Adequate energy and fatigue levels? 4. Gets around school environment adequately?	
I. Visual/Motor	
1. Uses age-appropriate grasp (pencils/crayons)? 2. Uses objects (scissors, erasers) with skill? 3. Draws/writes legibly with even force and spacing? 4. Uses dominant/assist hands appropriately?	

Impressions:
(Summarize observations, identify any further assessment needed, outline recommendations.)

School Observation: Environment*

Student observed:______________________________ Age:__________ Date: ________________

Activity:______________________________ Environment observed: ______________________________

The following questions help identify environmental factors that facilitate or interfere with learning. Observe all relevant spaces of the student's environment, such as classrooms, gym, cafeteria, bathrooms, playground, and hallways.

Observation of the General Environment

Room Arrangement	**Observations**
1. Room size and shape adequate for task?	Yes No
2. Furniture/equipment arrangement?	Diagram room on blank sheet
3. Varied space available?	Intimate 6″–18″ Personal 1½′ – 4′ Social 4′–12′
4. Space for personal belongings?	Describe:
5. Active and quiet spots?	Yes No

Traffic Patterns	
1. Clearly defined pathways?	Yes No
2. All areas and materials accessible?	Yes No
3. Any architectural barriers?	Yes No
4. Time and distance student covers:	Describe:

Routines	
1. Adequate structured/unstructured time?	Yes No
2. Toileting, drinks, snack?	As needed Scheduled

**Materials created by Barbara Hanft and Patricia Place.*

Observation of the Sensory Environment

Auditory	Observations
1. Sounds in and out of observed setting?	Describe:
2. Unique acoustical features?	Carpet Cinder block Other

Visual	
1. Adequate light?	Yes No Source: _____ Natural _____ Fixtures
2. How is color used?	Highlight Guide Background Other:
3. Intense glare on materials?	Yes No
4. Unique visual features?	Describe:

Tactile/Kinesthetic	
1. Flooring	Tile ______ % Carpet ______ % Other ______ %
2. Use of textures in furniture/materials?	Describe:
3. Light touch from others?	Describe:
4. Unique tactile features?	Describe:

Movement	
1. What movement/breaks are permitted?	Describe:
2. Who moves through this space and how efficiently?	Describe:
3. Unique movement features?	Describe:

Observation of a Particular Learning Environment

Intent of Space	Observations
1. What is this space intended to facilitate?	Learning, resting, playing? Fine motor, gross motor, language, academic, social, self-help? Independent, cooperative? Intent unclear?
2. Clear boundaries?	Yes No
3. Enough space?	Yes No
4. Necessary materials easily accessible?	Yes No
5. Materials/furniture enhance performance?	Yes No
6. Time student is seated and/or in same position?	Time: ______ Seated ______ Same position

Recommendations for improving student performance:

School Consultation Plan*

Student's name: ______________________ Age: ________ Date: ______________

Collaborators: ______________________ Role: ______________________

______________________ Role: ______________________

______________________ Role: ______________________

1. When and where the consulting therapist will observe/assess/work with the student:

Dates:	Where (classroom, PE, lunch, recess, bathroom, other)?

2. When the consulting therapist will meet with team members for planning:

Dates:	Who? At what time?

3. Student's strengths (observed by educational team and consulting therapist):

4. Student's functional problems (observed by educational team and consulting therapist):

**Materials created by Barbara Hanft and Patricia Place.*

5. Student's desired educational outcomes (describe desired performance/behavior):

6. Recommendations for intervention:

What to try:	Who will do it?	When?

7. Follow-up plan

How will consulting therapist follow up?	When?

Consultant Skills Inventory*

This inventory can help you identify your areas of competence as a consultant as well as pinpoint areas for improvement. Rate your level of skill for each of the items below according to the following scale:

A: *I need to improve this skill.* **B: *I perform this skill adequately.*** **C: *I perform this skill very well.***

Interpersonal Skills	A	B	C
1. I communicated clearly and avoided professional jargon.			
2. I used active listening skills, such as paraphrasing, clarifying, and summarizing, to facilitate the consultation process.			
3. I understood the tasks and responsibilities for each team member.			
4. I elicited team member's observations and viewpoints.			
5. I enabled others to examine their viewpoints of a situation or stated problem and to consider other possible views or explanations.			
6. I managed conflict skillfully and mediated between team members when necessary.			
7. I reinforced and supported the efforts of other team members.			
Collaborative Problem Solving			
1. I identified and clarified problems and needs with team members.			
2. I used a team approach to identify common goals and intervention strategies for the student's educational program.			
3. I used collaborative brainstorming to generate potential solutions to problems and strategies to accomplish objectives.			
4. I integrated feasible alternatives into my consultation plan.			
5. I elicited information to evaluate the effectiveness of the planned educational intervention.			
6. I encouraged the team to reconsider, if necessary, and to change interventions.			
7. I provided information from my own area of expertise without overwhelming others and while acknowledging others' expertise.			
Professional Development			
1. I was able to assess my own effectiveness from the student's progress, parental and staff feedback, and my own self-perceptions.			
2. I requested and accepted feedback and suggestions for improvement.			
3. I sought professional development through conferences, workshops, meetings, or individual study and reading.			

*Adapted with permission from: Klein, S., and S. Kontos. 1993. Best Practices in Integration (BPI) Inservice Training Model. Bloomington, IN: Indiana University.

Notes on my progress and successes:

Goals:

References

American Occupational Therapy Association. 1991a. *Essentials and guidelines for an accredited program for occupational therapists*. Bethesda, MD: AOTA.

American Occupational Therapy Association. 1991b. *Essentials and guidelines for an accredited program for certified occupational therapy assistants*. Bethesda, MD: AOTA.

American Occupational Therapy Association. 1993. *1993 member data survey*. Bethesda, MD: AOTA.

American Occupational Therapy Association Pediatric Task Force. 1989. *Survey of pediatric occupational therapy entry level practice and education*. Bethesda, MD: AOTA.

American Physical Therapy Association. 1994. *1993 active membership profile report*. Alexandria, VA: APTA.

Apter, D. 1994. From dream to reality: A participant's view of the implementation of Part H of P.L. 99-457. *Journal of Early Intervention* 18(2):131-140.

Ayres, A. 1979. *Sensory integration and the child*. Los Angeles: Western Psychological.

Babcock, N., and W. Pryzwansky. 1983. Models of consultation: Preferences of educational professionals at five stages of service. *Journal of School Psychology* 21:359-366.

Benson, S. 1993. Collaborative teaming: A model for occupational therapists working in inclusive schools. *Developmental Disabilities Special Interest Newsletter* 16(4):1-4.

Bergan, J., and A. Neumann. 1980. The identification of resources and constraints influencing plan design in consultation. *Journal of School Psychology* 18:317-323.

Bergan, J., and M. Tombari. 1976. Consultant skill and efficiency and the implementation and outcomes of consultation. *Journal of School Psychology* 14:3-14.

Board of Education v. Rowley, 458 U.S. 176, 102 S. CT. 3034, 73 L. Ed., 2d 690 (1982).

Bronfenbrenner, U. 1977. Toward an experimental ecology of human development. *American Psychologist* 32:513-531.

Brown, D., M. Wyne, J. Blackburn, and W. Powell. 1979. *Consultation: Strategy for improving education*. Boston: Allyn and Bacon.

Bundy, A. 1991. Consultation and sensory integration theory. In *Sensory integration: Theory and practice*, 317-332. Edited by A. Fisher, E. Murray, and A. Bundy. Philadelphia: F. A. Davis.

Campbell, P., W. McInerney, and M. Cooper. 1984. Therapeutic programming for students with severe handicaps. *American Journal of Occupational Therapy* 38(9):594-602.

Chandler, B. 1992. *How to design and implement classroom programming*. In *Classroom applications for school-based practice*, edited by C. Royeen, Lesson 3. Bethesda, MD: American Occupational Therapy Association.

Chandler, B., W. Dunn, and J. Rourk. 1989. *Guidelines for occupational therapy services in the school systems*, 2d ed. Bethesda, MD: American Occupational Therapy Association.

Clark, G., and L. Porsch. 1993. Inclusive programming model: Making a dream a reality. *Developmental Disabilities Special Interest Newsletter* 16(4):4-5.

Cole, K., S. Harris, S. Eland, and P. Mills. 1989. Comparison of two service delivery models: In-class and out-of-class therapy approaches. *Pediatric Physical Therapy* 1:49-54.

Curtis, M., and J. Meyers. 1988. Consultation: A foundation for alternative services in the schools. In *Alternative educational delivery systems: Enhancing instructional options for all students*, edited by J. Graden, J. Zins, and M. Curtis. Washington, DC: National Association for School Psychologists.

Dettmer, P., L. Thurston, and N. Dyck. 1993. *Consultation, collaboration and teamwork for students with special needs*. Boston: Allyn and Bacon.

Dunn, W. 1990. A comparison of service-provision models in school-based occupational therapy services: A pilot study. *Occupational Therapy Journal of Research* 10(5):300-320.

Dunn, W. 1991. Consultation as a process: How, when and why? In *School-based practice for related services,* edited by C. Royeen. Rockville, MD: American Occupational Therapy Association.

Dunn, W., and P. Campbell. 1991. Designing pediatric service provision. In *Pediatric occupational therapy: Facilitating effective service provision,* edited by W. Dunn. Thorofare, NJ: Slack.

Edmondson, K., and J. Spell. 1991. Written materials and the client with low literacy skills. *Infants and Young Children* 4(1):62-67.

Education for All Handicapped Children Act of 1975. U.S. Public Law 94-142. 20th Congress. 1975.

Education for the Handicapped Law Report. Horsham, PA: LRP.

Effgen, S. 1988. Preparation of physical and occupational therapists to work in early childhood special education settings. *Topics in Early Childhood Special Education* 7(4):10-19.

Effgen, S. 1994. The educational environment. In *Physical Therapy for Children.* Edited by S. Campbell, R. Palisano, and D. Vanderlinden. Philadelphia: Saunders.

Feinberg, E. Personal communication. 15 November 1994.

Fisher, J. 1994. Physical therapy in educational environments: Moving through time with reflections and visions. *Pediatric Physical Therapy* 6(3):144-147.

Fisher, R., and W. Ury. 1983. *Getting to yes.* New York: Penguin Books.

Gallesich, J. 1982. *The profession and practice of consultation.* San Francisco: Jossey-Bass.

Giangreco, M. 1986. Effects of integrated therapy: A pilot study. *Journal of the Association for Persons with Severe Handicaps* 6:15-21.

Gilfoyle, E., and C. Hays, Eds. 1980. *Training occupational therapy educational management in the schools (TOTEMS).* Bethesda, MD: American Occupational Therapy Association.

Glidewell, J. 1959. The entry problem in consultation. *Journal of Social Issues* 15:51-59.

Gordon, J., R. Zemke, and P. Jones, Eds. 1981. *Designing and delivering cost-effective training.* Minneapolis: Lakewood.

Hanft, B. 1989. Early intervention: Issues in specialization. *American Journal of Occupational Therapy* 43(7):431-434.

Hanft, B., and J. Burke. 1993. *Narrative interview: Understanding the family story.* Workshop presentation, AOTA Annual Conference, Boston, July 7.

Hanft, B., and J. Thomas. 1995. Evolution and revolution: David is growing up. *Developmental Disabilities Special Interest Section* 18(1):1-3.

Hanft, B., J. Burke, M. Cahill, K. Swenson-Miller, and R. Humphry. 1992. *Working with families: A curriculum guide for pediatric occupational therapists.* Chapel Hill, NC: Frank Porter Graham Child Development Center, University of North Carolina.

Hildebrand, V. 1971. *Introduction to early childhood education.* New York: Macmillan.

Idol, L. 1988. A rationale and guidelines for establishing special education consultation programs. *Remedial and Special Education* 9(6):48-57.

Idol, L., A. Nevin, and P. Paolucci-Whitcomb. 1994. *Collaborative consultation,* 2d ed. Austin, TX: PRO-ED.

Idol, L., P. Paolucci-Whitcomb, and A. Nevin. 1987. *Collaborative consultation.* Austin, TX: PRO-ED.

Idol, L., and J. West. 1987. Consultation in special education (part II): Training and practice. *Journal of Learning Disabilities* 20(8):474-493.

Idol-Maestas, L. 1983. *Special educator's consultation handbook.* Rockville, MD: Aspen.

Idol-Maestas, L., and A. Ritter. 1985. A follow-up study of resource/consulting teachers. *Teacher Education and Special Education* 8(3):121-131.

Individuals with Disabilities Education Act. Public Law 101-476 (Chapter 33). 20th Congress.

Johnson, J., M. Pugach, and D. Hammittee. 1988. Barriers to effective special education consultation. *Remedial and Special Education* 9(6):41-47.

Klein, D. 1976. Some notes on the dynamics of resistance to change: The defender role. In *The planning of change,* edited by W. Bennis, K. Benne, R. Chin, and K. Corey, 117-124. New York: Holt, Rinehart and Winston.

Klein, S., and S. Kontos. 1993. *Best practices in integration (BPI) inservice training model.* Bloomington, IN: Indiana University.

Knoff, H., A. McKenna, and K. Riser. 1991. Toward a consultant effectiveness scale: Investigating the characteristics of effective consultants. *School Psychology Review* 20:81-96.

Komich, P. Personal communication. 16 October 1991.

Kramer, S. 1992. A "snapshot" and "developing picture." In *Working with families: A curriculum guide for pediatric occupational therapists* by B. Hanft, J. Burke, M. Cahill, K. Swenson-Miller, and R. Humphry. Chapel Hill, NC: University of North Carolina. (Frank Porter Graham Child Development Center, CB#8180, UNC Campus, Chapel Hill, NC 27599-8180)

Lillie, D., and P. Place. 1982. *Partners: A guide to working with schools for parents of children with special instructional needs.* Glenview, IL: Scott, Foresman.

Lippitt, G., and R. Lippitt. 1978. *The consulting process in action.* San Diego: University Associates.

The living Webster encyclopedic dictionary of the English language. Chicago: The English Language Institute of America.

Lynch, E., and M. Hanson. 1992. *Developing cross-cultural competence.* Baltimore: Paul H. Brookes.

Marris, P. 1986. *Loss and change.* London: Routledge Kegan Paul.

Martin, K., Ed. 1990. *Physical therapy practice in educational environments,* 2d ed. Alexandria, VA: American Physical Therapy Association.

McCormack, G. 1987. Culture and communication in the treatment planning for occupational therapy with minority patients. *Occupational Therapy in Health Care* 4(1):17-36.

McGlothlin, M., and D. Kelly. 1982. Issues facing the resource teacher. *Learning Disability Quarterly* 5:58-64.

Medway, F., and J. Updyke. 1985. Metanalysis of consultation outcome studies. *American Journal of Community Psychology* 13(4):489-505.

Merriam, S., and P. Cunningham. 1989. *Handbook of adult and continuing education.* San Francisco: Jossey Bass.

Meyers, J., L. Gelzheiser, and R. Yelich. 1991. Do pull-in programs foster teacher collaboration? *Remedial and Special Education* 12(2):7-15.

Miller, T., and D. Sabatino. 1978. An evaluation of the teacher consultation model as an approach to mainstreaming. *Exceptional Children* 45(2):86-91.

Mills v. DC Board of Education, 348 F. Supp. 866 (D.D.C. 1972); contempt proceedings, EHLR 551:643 (D.D.C. 1980).

Mitchell, D., and S. Tucker. 1992. Leadership as a way of thinking. *Educational Leadership* 49(5):30-35.

Neel, R. 1981. How to put the consultant to work in consulting teaching. *Behavioral Disorders* 6(2):78-81.

Palisano, R. 1989. Comparison of two methods of service delivery for students with learning disabilities. *Physical and Occupational Therapy in Pediatrics* 9(3):79-99.

Peck, C., C. Killen, and D. Baumgart. 1989. Increasing implementation of special education instruction in mainstream preschools: Direct and generalized nondirective consultation. *Journal of Applied Behavioral Analysis* 22:197-210.

Pennsylvania Association for Retarded Children (PARC) v. Commonwealth of Pennsylvania, 334 F. Supp. 1257, 279 (E.D. Pa. 1971, 1972).

Phillips, V., and L. McCullough. 1990. Consultation-based programming: Instituting the collaborative ethic in schools. *Exceptional Children* 56(4):291-304.

Pryzwansky, W., and G. White. 1983. The influence of consultee characteristics on preferences for consultation approaches. *Professional Psychology: Research and Practice* 14:457-461.

Rainforth, B., J. York, and C. MacDonald. 1992. *Collaborative teams for students with severe disabilities*. Baltimore: Paul H. Brookes.

Rogers, E. 1983. *Diffusion of innovation,* 3d ed. New York: The Free Press.

Rose, P. 1970. *The study of society.* New York: Random House.

Royeen, C., Ed. 1991. *School-based practice for related services.* Bethesda, MD: American Occupational Therapy Association.

Royeen, C., Ed. 1992. *Classroom applications for school-based practice.* Bethesda, MD: American Occupational Therapy Association.

Schowengerdt, R., M. Fine, and J. Poggio. 1976. An examination of some bases of teacher satisfaction with school psychological services. *Psychology in the Schools* 13:269-275.

Schulte, A., S. Osborne, and J. McKinney. 1990. Academic outcomes for students with learning disabilities in consultation and resource programs. *Exceptional Children* 57(2):162-172.

Spake, E. 1994. Reflections and visions: The state of pediatric curricula. *Pediatric Physical Therapy* 6(3):128-132.

Sparling, J. 1992. *A guide for embedding family information into an entry-level physical therapy curriculum.* Chapel Hill, NC: Frank Porter Graham Child Development Center, University of North Carolina.

Speece, D., and C. Mandell. 1980. Resource room support services for regular teachers. *Learning Disability Quarterly* 3:49-53.

Stainback, S., and W. Stainback. 1985. The merger of special and regular education: Can it be done? A response to Lieberman and Mesinger. *Exceptional Children* 51(6):517-521.

Sweeney, J., C. Heriza, and R. Markowitz. 1994. The changing profile of pediatric physical therapy: A 10-year analysis of clinical practice. *Pediatric Physical Therapy* 6(3):113-118.

Turnbull, H. R. 1986. *Free appropriate public education: The law and children with disabilities.* Denver: Love.

Ury, W. 1993. *Getting past no.* New York: Bantam Books.

Weisbourd, M. 1992. *Discovering common ground.* San Francisco: Berrett-Koehler.

Weissenburger, J., M. Fine, and J. Poggio. 1982. The relationship of selected consultant/teacher characteristics to consultation outcomes. *Journal of School Psychology* 20:263-270.

West, J., and G. Cannon. 1988. Essential collaborative consultation competencies for regular and special educators. *Journal of Learning Disabilities* 21:56-63.

Will, M. 1988. Letter to Mary Jo Butler re: physical and occupational therapy in the schools. *Education for the Handicapped Law Report* Supplement 215, April 22:118-121.

York, J., B. Rainforth, and M. Giangreco. 1990. Transdisciplinary teamwork and integrated therapy: Clarifying some misperceptions. *Pediatric Physical Therapy* 2(2):73-79.

School System

Special Interest Section Quarterly

Volume 9, Number 1 • March 2002

Published by the American Occupational Therapy Association, Inc.

A Collaborative Partnership: Creating Developmentally Appropriate Teaching Practices for Pre-K and Kindergarten

■ Heidi B. Schoenfeld MA, OTR; Patricia Mesquiti, MA

Staff development for teachers who teach students with disabilities yet who work primarily outside of the area of special education has been mandated both in the Individuals With Disabilities Education Act Reauthorization of 1997 (Public Law 105–17) (Heumann & Hehir, 1997; Muhlenhaupt, Miller, Sanders, & Swinth, 1998) and in Texas State Law (Texas Education Agency, 2001, § 21.451). However, since its inception in 1989, the Northside Independent School District (NISD) Occupational Therapy Program has trained regular education teachers and staff members who work with special education students as an integral part of service delivery. Because many occupational therapy referrals are for handwriting difficulties, teachers are offered both formal and informal in-service training. Training includes information on the normal developmental sequence of readiness skill acquisition, activities that would facilitate skill development, and strategies for accommodating learner differences. This information is often overlooked in pre-service teacher education curriculum. As a last resort for students who cannot participate successfully in the district's adopted curriculum teachers receive instruction in an alternate handwriting program, Handwriting Without Tears TM (HWT) (Olsen, 1998). The HWT program is a developmentally based sequence of systematic instruction. Over the years, many of the teachers have found that the strategies used with their students with special needs from the alternative handwriting program were applicable to teaching all children. Many teachers voiced dismay with the district curriculum, believing the alternate curriculum to be "student friendly" and able to produce better results. Teaching staff often questioned why the distrit did not adopt a handwriting curriculum that could meet the needs of our diverse learners. We had a dual curriculum. Should not *all* children have access to and benefit from "best practices?"

With the emphasis on standards, accountability, and high stakes testing, teachers and administrators have been forced to add more content to the already-full curriculum. Politicians and parents have clamored that reading and writing should be taught at an earlier age in hopes that this will prepare children to pass the tests. Occupational therapists know, though, that a normal sequence exists to the development of prerequisite skills required for the higher-order thinking needed for academics, such as reading and writing (Ayres, 1987; Bredekamp, 1992; Weil & Amundson, 1994).

Allowances for the natural processes of growth and development and early experiences are paramount to academic success. Expecting children to perform activities such as writing before acquiring the prerequisite skills can lead to a cycle of failure. Frustration, tension, poor self-esteem, and withdrawal from the activity may cause the child to resist participating in the activity, even when developmentally ready (Landry & Burridge, 1999). Therefore, professionals who work with young children must articulate what is best practice and educate the stakeholders that providing what is appropriate for young children can facilitate desired future outcomes.

This article describes a collaborative partnership between the NISD lead occupational therapist and the instructional specialist for the pre-k and kindergarten programs. The partnership was forged for the purpose of creating developmentally appropriate teaching practices and curriculum for young children.

Academics 2000 Project

In keeping with the district's mission (statement of beliefs and goals) and strategic plan, the NISD Department of Elementary Instruction applied for and was awarded an Academics 2000 grant. The state funds for this grant came from the federal Goals 2000 monies allocated to the states. In the spring of 1995, Academics 2000 was launched to develop a language arts curriculum for the early primary grades (pre-k through second grade). The *Primary Early Learning Framework* (PELF) was the result of a 3-year project.

Patricia Mesquiti, pre-k and kindergarten instructional specialist, was charged with coordinating and facilitating the Academics 2000 project. She noticed a disconnection between student learning/performance expectations and developmental readiness. Familiar with the role of occupational therapy in NISD and having worked with Heidi Schoenfeld, Lead Occupational Therapist, on mutual district committees, Mesquiti asked Schoenfeld to attend the initial Academics 2000 planning session in the spring of 1995. After the plans were under way to form committees, Mesquiti believed Schoenfeld's knowledge and expertise would best be served on the subcommittee charged with looking at the continuum of writing.

For the next 2 years, collaborative team of early learning teaching experts, with various backgrounds and experiences, and the lead occupational therapist tackled the daunting task of developing standards for diverse learners and creating developmentally appropriate and effective teaching practices. When implemented, these standards and practices will align with the state standards. Lastly, this framework must link to the continuum of skills designed to enable the student to pass the high stakes administered in upper grades.

The occupational therapist provided a new prospective to the team. With a strong background in normal child development and expertise in handwriting, the teachers looked to her for guidance in understanding the developmental prerequisites for writing and the connection between penmanship and language composition. When determining the most effective teaching practices, discussions regard-

ing careful consideration of each child's developmental level and needs were critical. The committee decided that the final document must include information on normal hand and visual-motor development as well as information on remedial activities and compensatory strategies for students who are acquiring skills at a slower rate. Information regarding the consideration of the student's level of arousal and simple adaptation to materials was included. As a result, sections in the final document include information on age-appropriate activities for young children in a school setting that facilitate the development of foundational skills and lead to academic success. Some examples of resources in the document recommended by the occupational therapist are (a) a list of specific activities designed to improve hand strength and dexterity using materials typically found in the early learning classrooms; (b) suggested techniques to facilitate a functional pencil grasp, including a diagram of functional and dysfunctional pencil grasp patterns, and information about the variety of writing implements and pencil grips; (c) visual-motor and prewriting activities, including the diagram of requisite strokes and age norm equivalencies developed by Beery and Buktenica (Beery, 1997) and (d) a suggested sequence of letter introduction that is based on first introducing the easiest-to-form letters.

The teachers were able to share how the writing process influences success in all areas of academic work. Information about the diverse learners in their classes and the basic needs that must be met before students are ready to do academic tasks were explained. The subcommittee recognized the demands and limitations that affect the classroom teachers' ability to implement writing lessons that meet the needs of each child in the class. However, the committee believed that the document must equip the classroom teachers with some basic tools and information that would help them select the most appropriate activities and teaching strategies. In general, educators could assess the student's skill level and pick an activity or teaching approach from the continuum and array of ideas.

Outcomes of the Academics 2000 Project

In the fall of 1998, a comprehensive document, *Northside ISD Primary Early Learning Framework* (NISD, 1998), was distributed to all elementary campuses. The PELF was the result of a 3-year project. The PELF includes the following: (a) NISD standards for language arts, which align with state standards; (b) effective teaching practices for the oral language, reading, and writing continuums; (c) connection to the Texas Assessment of Academic Skills (the state-mandated test); and (d) content area applications. This document is the basis for student assessment, instructional decisions, and parent communication (NISD, 1998).

After the completion and distribution of the PELF, NISD occupational therapists were available on their assigned campuses to team with teaching and support staff members, consult with administrators, educate parents, and provide both informal and formal staff development.

The NISD occupational therapists are able to provide the staff development and support because they have flexibility to prioritize their workloads on the basis of campus needs. Workloads include collaborating with team members to develop individualized education programs (IEPs); attending conferences, staffings, annual reviews, transition and triennial meetings; and working with students in their school environments (off campus, if needed). The aforementioned activities are all part of the services provided on behalf of students and are stipulated in our annual reports and recommendations to the annual review committees (IEP meeting). Time and frequency for occupational therapy services are indicated on the IEP as blocks of minutes per year, giving therapists the ability to address needs as they arise rather than on an arbitrary, preset schedule. Staff development may take place through informal meetings with teachers and support staff members or through structured workshops. Both campus-specific and district-wide staff development offerings are provided. One of our most successful training modules is scheduling a day on one campus where teachers attend a session during their scheduled conference time with their grade-level team. This arrangement has allowed the therapist to tailor the handwriting in-service to the needs of a smaller, more homogeneous group. Teaching staff members have been more likely to integrate the information into the classroom with this type of training. The therapist is available for follow-up questions, and the training has resulted in the reduction of referrals for occupational therapy evaluation and service delivery to address handwriting concerns.

Forging a Shared Vision

Stakeholders began to see the link between the language component and the mechanics of writing and understand that the ability to write begins long before children hold a pencil in their hand. We, the authors, realized that if NISD children were to be afforded the best early education experience that would prepare them for future academic challenges, the work started with the Academics 2000 initiative needed to continue. The adopted handwriting program for NISD needed revisiting; the pre-k and kindergarten teachers needed to include more developmentally appropriate activities before beginning more structured writing activities; and more formal teaching staff development opportunities to address developmentally appropriate practices were essential. We had forged a partnership and a shared vision.

The Handwriting Without Tears™ (HWT) program (Olsen, 1998) continued to be recommended for students with special needs who are not participating successfully in the adopted handwriting curriculum. The staff occupational therapists instruct teachers on the program, providing suggestions for "warm-up" activities and recommending prewriting activities for those students not ready for formal instruction. Several years ago, the district administration agreed to allow teachers to incorporate HWT strategies in general education enabling more students to successfully form letters. However, the present NISD adopted curriculum would remain.

In 1999, the Texas State Board of Education approved the HWT curriculum for use in Texas schools. We, the authors, realized that implementing new programs often meet with some resistance. We also thought that introducing a new handwriting curriculum at a time when teachers were already faced with other district-wide changes would not be popular. We proposed to the elementary program administration a pilot program for implementation at the pre-k and kindergarten level on campuses with teachers demonstrating interest in the curriculum. The response was initially positive; however, as time for training drew near, a change in circumstances required a change in plans: Including the kindergarten program for the 2001–2002 school year would not be feasible. It was possible, however, to hold an in-service for all pre-k teaching staff members on developmentally appropriate practices (in terms of prewriting) as part of the language and literacy training component.

Faced with new challenges and constraints, the authors decided to begin with staff development for the pre-k teachers regarding the sequential requisites for the development of writing readiness skills. Based on the premise that opportunity for movement and experimental play build a strong foundation for higher thinking (Bredekamp, 1992), the goal of the training provided by the occupational therapy staff would be to help the teachers gain an understanding of the motor and behavioral skills required for later academic success. Teachers would gain insight into activity analysis, and specific developmental activities would be shared. The HWT curriculum also would be introduced. Although formal handwriting instruction is discouraged in pre-k, introducing some of the prewriting activities, such as using the readiness materials, was appropriate. Familiarizing teachers

SCHOOL SYSTEM

SPECIAL INTEREST SECTION QUARTERLY

(ISSN 1093-7242)

Published quarterly by The American Occupational Therapy Association, Inc., 4720 Montgomery Lane, Bethesda, MD 20814-3425; ajotsis@aota.org (e-mail). Periodicals postage paid at Bethesda, MD. POSTMASTER: Send address changes to *School System Special Interest Section Quarterly*, AOTA, PO Box 31220, Bethesda, MD 20824-1220. Annual membership dues are $187 for OTs, $111 for OTAs, and $53 for OT students. Special Interest Section (SIS) membership, including a subscription to the *SIS Quarterly*, for OTs and OTAs is $25 for the first and $15 for each additional. SIS membership for students is $10 for the first and $5 for each additional. Nonmembers may subscribe to the *SIS Quarterly(s)* of their choice for $50 each per year. The opinions and positions stated by the contributors are those of the authors and not necessarily those of the editor or AOTA.

Chairperson: Yvonne Swinth
Editor: Sue Ann DuBois
Managing Editor: Barbara Scanlan

with the HWT printing program would allow them to show students who have readiness skills and are experimenting with print how to form letters correctly.

The initial training was scheduled for June 2001 as part of the weeklong summer staff development opportunity that NISD offers each year. The training session included teachers from the PPCD. At NISD, the PPCD teachers team with the pre-k teachers because many of the students with special needs spend all or part of their instructional day in the pre-k or kindergarten classroom. HWT manuals and readiness materials were available for each teacher attending the workshop. Response was positive; a follow-up for those receiving the training was scheduled for September 2001. Teachers unable to attend the summer training were required to attend a fall session, with follow-up in January 2002. The staff occupational therapist assigned to each campus is available for consultation throughout the year.

The authors' long-term goal is that all primary grades utilize the HWT program. This would involve more collaborative partners. Many of our students with special needs already use the HWT program. Adopting HWT as a district-wide curriculum will eliminate a dual system for handwriting instruction and facilitate all children learning together.

Lessons Learned

It took many years before that dream was realized, and the following lessons were learned. First and foremost, be aware that dreams are not realized overnight. Baby steps may be necessary. Second, find kindred souls and "dream and scheme" together. The more persons you involve, the more likely an idea will be talked about and considered. Third, be flexible and open-minded. You may need to weather change in plans, a turn in the road, or more time before your ideas can get off the ground. Fourth, be steadfast; modify but do not give up when faced with adversity. Look for other opportunities and go forth. Finally and most importantly, keep dreaming. There always are new heights to climb, and remember that you will need a partner while hiking up the mountain.

Summary

We hope that this article will inspire you to think outside of the box. Working in today's schools is challenging, to say the least. There are many more job requirements than time allotted to meet the demands adequately. Often, it is easier to continue to perform the job in the same familiar manner, even when faced with change, but in the end, this will not work. Therapists in schools must continue to face the growing demands with effective and efficient solutions. Many more children can be affected positively when you make system changes. You may need to form new partnerships. Stretch your imagination. Use your talents. "Team and scheme" for all the children. They are our future. ■

Acknowledgment

We thank Cheryl Horton, OTR, for her comments and editorial skills.

References

Ayres, A. J. (1987). *Sensory integration and the child.* Los Angeles: Western Psychological Services.

Beery, K. E. (1997). The Beery-Buktenica Developmental Test of Visual-Motor Integration, 4th ed. Parsippany, NJ: Modern Curriculum Press.

Bredekamp, S. (Ed.). (1992). *Developmentally appropriate practice in early childhood programs serving children birth through age 8.* Washington DC: National Association for the Education of Young Children.

Heumann, J. E., & Hehir, T. (1997, September). Believing in children: A great IDEA for the future [Electronic version]. *Exceptional Parent.* (Article can be found at http://www.ed.gov/offices/OSEP/IDEA/article2.html

Individuals With Disabilities Education Act Reauthorization of 1997. Pub. L. 105–17, 20 U.S.C. § 1400 et seq.

Landry, J. M., & Burridge, K. R. (1999). *Fine motor skills and handwriting activities for young children.* West Nyack, NY: The Center for Applied Research in Education.

Muhlenhaupt, M., Miller, H., Sanders, J., & Swinth, Y. (1998, September). Implications of the 1997 reauthorization of IDEA for school-based occupational therapy. *School System Specialty Interest Section Quarterly, 5,* 1–4.

Northside Independent School District. (1998). *Northside ISD: Primary early learning framework.* (Available from Northside Independent School District, 5900 Evers Road, San Antonio, Texas 78238)

Northside Independent School District. (2000). *Welcome to Northside ISD.* (Available from Northside Independent School District, 5900 Evers Road, San Antonio, Texas 78238)

Olsen, J. Z. (1998). *Handwriting Without Tears.* (Available from Jan Z. Olsen, OTR, 8802 Quiet Stream Court, Potomac, Maryland 20854)

Texas Education Agency, Division of Special Education. (2001). *Special education rules and regulations.* (Texas Education Agency). Austin, TX: Author.

Weil, M. J., & Amundson, S. J. C., (1994). Relationship between visuomotor and handwriting skills of children in kindergarten. *American Journal of Occupational Therapy, 48,* 982–988.

***Heidi B. Schoenfeld**, MA, OTR, is Lead Occupational Therapist, Northside Independent School District, 4711 Sid Katz, San Antonio, Texas 78229, the SSSIS Chair for the Texas Occupational Therapy Association, and a member of the AOTA IDEA National Resource Cadre; HeidiSchoenfeld@nisd.net. **Patricia Mesquiti**, MA, is Pre-K and Kindergarten Instructional Specialist, Northside Independent School District, San Antonio, Texas, and is a member of the Association for Childhood Education International and the Association for Supervision and Curriculum Development.*

Schoenfeld, H. B., & Mesquiti, P. (2002, March). A collaborative partnership: Creating developmentally appropriate teaching practices for pre-k and kindergarten. *School System Special Interest Section Quarterly, 9,* 1–2, 4.

SS